# Caring for Kids

## Useful Information & Hard-to-Find Facts
## About Child Health & Development

Compliments Of:

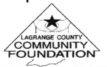

By Patricia A. Keener, M.D.

James Whitcomb Riley Memorial Association
Indianapolis, Indiana

# Dear Reader

I am proud to present to you a very special gift! As the state's only comprehensive children's hospital, Riley Hospital for Children has produced a book for anyone who cares for and about children. It is called *Caring for Kids*. The idea for the book came from the Riley Memorial Association, the fund-raising arm of the hospital.

After receiving funding from Lilly Endowment Inc., we sought the best writer for the project. Everyone involved was thrilled when Patricia A. Keener, M.D., Clinical Professor of Pediatrics at Indiana University School of Medicine, agreed to author the book. Her contributions to health education have been recognized with several prestigious national awards. She is also the founder and medical director of Safe Sitter, a national organization that teaches adolescents safe child care techniques.

With input and recommendations from physicians, health care professionals and parents throughout Indiana, Dr. Keener and her staff spent many hours making sure the book met our vision – it contains thousands of interesting facts, pages of useful information, and listings of resources meant for parents, grandparents, and care providers of children ages newborn to 21. It is divided into four useful sections: *Child Health Care, Growth and Development, Nutrition,* and *Child Safety*. The book is neither intended to be a comprehensive manual on child care nor to replace your doctor's instructional material. Instead, *Caring for Kids* is a supplement to this information and is meant to guide, inform and delight.

Please don't hesitate to tell your family, friends and neighbors about *Caring for Kids*. There are many ways for them to get the book, including logging on to Riley Memorial Association's Web site at *www.rileykids.org* or calling the Riley Memorial Association at (317) 634.4474.

I hope that you will find *Caring for Kids* to be a valuable resource.

Best regards,

*Richard L. Schreiner*

Richard L. Schreiner, M.D.
Chairman, Department of Pediatrics
Physician-in-Chief, Riley Hospital for Children

# How to Use this Book

*Caring for Kids* is divided into four sections. The final pages of each section contain resources, including helpful organizations, books, and Web sites.

## Section One: Child Health Care

This section begins with a brief history of child health care and childhood over the last 200 years. A detailed discussion of the well child visit is followed by brief discussions of dental and eye care. You will find information about sick child care, including when to keep your child home and how sick is sick.

## Section Two: Growth & Development

This section features interesting facts about growth and development beginning with the newborn and progressing through adolescence. You'll find discussions of physical growth, emotional development, important milestones, and age-related safety concerns. You will discover new insights into how your child's brain develops in "Brain Facts." The final pages of each age group are devoted to age-related safety concerns.

## Section Three: Nutrition

This section presents nutritional information for each developmental stage beginning with "Before Your Baby is Born" and proceeding through the teen years. Information on "Fat in Your Child's Diet" and "What Parents Should Know about Vegetarian Diets" conclude this section.

## Section Four: Child Safety

This section covers common childhood injuries and provides practical pointers for keeping your family safe. Use the "Home Safety Checklist" with the "Room-by-Room Checklist" to make sure your home is a safe home.

# Acknowledgements

The original idea to produce a handbook of practical health care information for families with children ages newborn to 21 was that of the Riley Memorial Association, the fund-raising arm of Riley Hospital for Children. The many tasks required to move this idea from concept to reality were accomplished by the dedicated staff of the Riley Memorial Association. Generous funding from Lilly Endowment Inc. makes it possible to provide *Caring for Kids* as a gift to every household in Indiana.

Richard L. Schreiner, M.D., the Chairman of the Department of Pediatrics at the Indiana University School of Medicine and Physician-in-Chief at Riley Hospital for Children, provided the encouragement and support critical to the completion of this manuscript.

## Author

Patricia A. Keener, M.D., Clinical Professor of Pediatrics at Indiana University School of Medicine, developed the concept and authored the text for *Caring for Kids*. Her contributions to health education for the general public have been recognized by several prestigious state and national awards, including the State of Indiana, Sagamore of the Wabash, and the Ross Award for Lay Education given by the American Academy of Pediatrics. Dr. Keener is founder and medical director of Safe Sitter, a national non-profit organization that teaches young adolescents safe and nurturing child care techniques. Dr. Keener's work with children's programming is partially supported by a grant from Reilly Foundation.

## Special thanks to the following experts:

*Caring for Kids* benefited from the thoughtful input and technical review of a number of individuals. James Cumming, M.D., reviewed the material from the perspective of a practicing pediatrician, knowledgeable about child health and primary care practice. Philip Merk, M.D., reviewed the manuscript from the perspective of a primary care physician in academic practice in a public hospital. The following physicians or health care professionals acted in the role of content experts: Margaret Blythe, M.D.; Sue Brady, DMSc, RD,

CSP; James Lemons, M.D.; and Karyl Rickard, Ph.D., RD, CSP.
In addition, special thanks to Toya Corbitt, M.D., for her advice
and comments at an early stage of the manuscript and to Doris
Merritt, M.D., for her valuable input related to organization
and presentation.

## Special thanks to research assistants and creative advisors:

Molly Bozic was the key collaborator in the production of this
manuscript. Without her technical ability with computer
formatting, her keen interest in the field of pediatrics, her
knowledge and skills with the English language, her willingness
to work through weekends and vacations, combined with her
enthusiasm for the project, this manuscript in its present form
would not be possible.

The earliest participants in the creative process, manuscript
design, and technical research were a team of five talented,
bright, enthusiastic interns working in the office of Dr. Keener.
These five good-hearted souls, all of whom are preparing for
application to medical school, devoted many hours to poring
through textbooks, child care manuals, magazines, Web sites,
and informational brochures in search of "useful information
and hard-to-find facts." The book could not exist without
them: Allison Boester, Molly Bozic, Gracie Carver, Mary
Palecek, and Nikki Silver. In addition, Shirley Lawson and
Nancy Singleton cheerfully and competently supported the
project, performing "other duties as required."

## Special thanks to lay reviewers:

The following individuals served as lay reviewers and
advisors when the manuscript was a work-in-progress:
Kristina Keener Yeager, Janice Hicks-Slaughter, Sheila Hyatt,
Steve and Venita Kirchhoff, Jane Nitz, Doris Peck, Beth
Waters-Finston, Don and Marcia Bozic, and Keener Family
members Gerald, Leslie, and Nick.

# References

The primary references for this book include: Behrman RE, Kliegman RM, Jenson HB. *Nelson Textbook of Pediatrics* (2000). Green M, Palfrey J, eds. *Bright Futures: Guidelines for Health Supervision of Infants, Children, and Adolescents* (2000). Four books from the American Academy of Pediatrics: *Caring for Your Baby and Young Child: Birth to Age 5* (1991); *Caring for Your School-Age Child: Ages 5 to 12* (1995); *Caring for Your Adolescent: Ages 12 to 21* (1991); and *Guide to Your Child's Symptoms* (1997).

For specific sections, the primary references are as follows. Growth and Development – Levine MD, Carey WB, Crocker AC, eds. *Developmental – Behavioral Pediatrics,* (1999); three books from Brilliant Beginnings: *Baby Brain Basics: Birth to 12 Months* (2000); *Toddler Brain Basics: 12 to 24 Months* (2000); *Toddler Next Steps: 24 to 36 Months* (2000); Nutrition – American Academy of Pediatrics: *Guide to Your Child's Nutrition* (1999); Safety – National SAFE KIDS Campaign, Brandenburg, M. *Child Safe: A Practical Guide for Preventing Injuries;* American Academy of Pediatrics: *Injury Prevention and Control for Children and Youth* (1997).

# Section 1: Child Health Care

# Section 2: Growth & Development

# Section 3: Nutrition

# Section 4: Child Safety

# Child Health Care

## Section One

## In this Section:

- First-Aid Supplies
- Well Child Visits
- Immunization Info
- How Sick is Sick?
- When to Keep Your Child Home
- And Much More...

Did you ever wonder why kids get shots for diseases you've never heard of? Or why a 6-month-old's appointment with the doctor for an ear infection doesn't count for the 6-month well child visit?

Why see a dentist for a tooth that's going to fall out anyway? What is the normal blood pressure for a 3-year-old? Or a 10-year-old? Do kids have problems with high blood pressure?

In the *Child Health Care* section, you'll find the answers to these questions as well as lots of other useful information and hard-to-find facts on child health.

# First Aid

## Home First-Aid Kit
### Important Reminders

- Enroll in a first-aid and CPR (cardiopulmonary resuscitation) course. You should also be trained in CPR for infants. See "Choking – Be Ready to Rescue" in the *Child Safety* section.

- Prepare two first-aid kits, one for home and one for travel.

- Include a first-aid chart complete with written instructions for CPR in each kit. For information on how to obtain a first-aid chart, see "Choking – Be Ready to Rescue" in the *Child Safety* section.

- Store home first-aid supplies in a locked box or locked closet. Store travel first-aid kit in locked trunk or locked glove compartment.

- Tape emergency information card (see "Emergency Information" page 259) to the lid on the outside of the first-aid box.

- If any family member requires special medication for a life-threatening emergency, include that medication in each first-aid kit. For example, include injectable epinephrine for a child with a known life-threatening allergy to bee stings.

- If any family member has a medical condition that is likely to require special medicine, include that medication in each first-aid kit. For example, include an inhaler for a child with asthma.

- Tape a supply list to the inside of the lid. Write the date the kit was assembled or last checked. Beside each medication, write the expiration date. Replace medications before they expire. Replace all other supplies immediately after use.

# First-Aid Kit Contents

- ✔ Adhesive bandages – assorted sizes
- ✔ Nonstick dressings – 4-inch squares
- ✔ Roll of gauze – 1- and 2-inch rolls
- ✔ Adhesive tape – 1-inch roll
- ✔ Butterfly bandages
- ✔ Elastic bandage – 3-inch roll (with safety pins)
- ✔ Packet of cotton swabs
- ✔ Roll of absorbent cotton
- ✔ Round-tipped scissors
- ✔ Tweezers
- ✔ Unbreakable, digital thermometer
- ✔ Children's acetaminophen tablets or liquid
- ✔ Antihistamine tablets or liquid
- ✔ Syrup of ipecac
- ✔ Antibiotic cream
- ✔ Calamine lotion
- ✔ Alcohol wipes
- ✔ Disposable gloves
- ✔ Flashlight
- ✔ FIRST-AID CHART

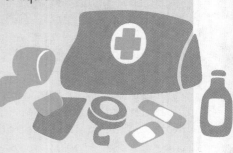

Source: American Academy of Pediatrics, *Guide to Your Child's Symptoms*

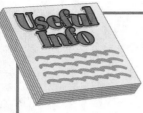

## Docs for Tots

Doctors began to specialize in the care of children in 1860. Before that, nurses or general doctors treated older children. Midwives or obstetricians treated children under 2.

Dr. Abraham Jacobi was the first physician in the United States to devote himself to the care of children. He is considered the *father of pediatrics in America*. In 1860 in New York, he established the first outpatient clinic for children.

Two years later in Paris, Dr. Pierre Budin, a French obstetrician, set up the first clinic for newborns. In addition to instructing parents in feeding and nutrition, he weighed and measured newborns – almost all of whom were born at home. Dr. Budin also established a nursery to care for sick newborns and premature babies.

## Show Time

In Paris, Dr. Budin became known for saving the lives of premature infants. One of the secrets of his success was to make sure the babies were kept comfortably warm. To provide warmth, Dr. Budin designed a simple machine called an incubator.

Hoping to interest the public in this new way to care for babies, Dr. Budin sent his student, Martin Couney, to the 1896 Berlin World Exposition with five premature infants, five incubators, and five nurses. People were very interested – up to 3,000 visitors a day filed by the tiny babies in their "human hatcheries!"

After Berlin, Couney traveled to various countries, including the United States, setting up his baby exhibits. As recently as 1939, the exhibit could be viewed at the New York World Fair.

# Lessons from the Past

A century ago, milk sold at the local store was dipped from an unrefrigerated five-gallon can. Very likely, molasses, chalk, or even plaster of Paris had been added to improve its taste or appearance. Infants and young children often became ill from the germs that thrived in the warm milk, especially in the summer months. At the time, infectious diseases 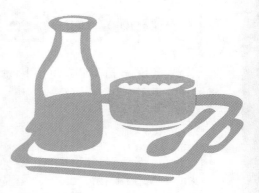 were the leading cause of death, and contaminated milk was a leading source of infection. The first major victory in the fight to save the lives of young children was won by setting standards for the safe handling of milks. "Milk stations" were set up where parents could get fresh milk from "certified" suppliers.

The next battle was fought against the killer diseases like diphtheria, tetanus, and pertussis (whooping cough). In the 1800s, these diseases filled graveyards with their tiny victims. Parents watched over their children as the disease ran its course to recovery or death. Doctors, called late in the disease when death was close, faced desperate situations. During his years of practice, Dr. Abraham Jacobi, the nation's first doctor for children, performed emergency surgery on more than 2,500 children dying of a blocked windpipe, the deadly complication of diphtheria. Though his heroic actions saved many children, tragically he was unable to save his own son. When the diphtheria vaccine became available, parents celebrated the chance to protect their children.

Development of the vaccine to prevent diphtheria was followed by vaccines for pertussis, tetanus, polio, measles, mumps – the list goes on to include more than a dozen childhood diseases that can be prevented by immunization. A parent of the 1800s would love to trade places with you. By having your child immunized, you can protect your child from diseases that once killed thousands of children.

# Child Health in the United States

## Live Healthier, Live Longer

- A child born in the year 2000 can expect to live to age 76. A child born in 1900 could have expected to live to age 50. Immunizations have made a major contribution to this gift of 26 extra years of life.

- Children who are immunized on schedule receive the maximum benefit from vaccines. In 1998, the immunization rate for young children 19 to 35 months of age was the highest ever recorded. Even so, 1 in every 4 children remains unprotected or only partially protected.

Source: U.S. Department of Health and Human Services

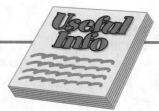

## What A Difference A Shot Makes

| Disease | Diphtheria | Measles | Pertussis | Paralytic Polio |
|---|---|---|---|---|
| **Before Vaccine** | | | | |
| Cases | 147,991 | 469,924 | 107,473 | 16,316 |
| Deaths | 13,170 | 7,575 | 5,099 | 1,879 |
| **After Vaccine** | | | | |
| Cases | 10 | 89 | 6,279 | 0 |
| Death | 1 | 0 | 9 | 0 |

Source: Centers for Disease Control & Prevention: *Achievements in Public Health, 1900-1999 Impact of Vaccines Universally Recommended for Children* – US, 1990-1998.

# Things Change

The 1800s were years of tremendous change in the United States. Thousands of families moved from small towns and farms to cities where factories offered employment. Factory-made clothing, furniture, and household items like soap and candles replaced handmade items. Middle-class women who could afford to purchase the factory-made goods had time available to spend with their children. Influenced by new ideas on childhood from Europe, these mothers directed their attention to educating their children using a far more gentle approach to parenting than past generations.

While children of middle- and upper-class families benefited from their parents' changing views on childhood, the children of the poor had no such advantage. Children as young as 7 worked long hours in low-paying jobs and were unable to take advantage of public education. The children in factories were not alone in their misfortune. The living conditions of orphanages were so terrible that only 1 of every 10 children placed in an orphanage was likely to survive. All children suffered from the problems of infectious disease and poor sanitation.

As the public became aware of the unhealthy and miserable conditions existing for children, public interest began to grow in the federal government's role in improving the welfare of children. In 1909, the first White House Conference on Children brought together social leaders, educators, doctors, and civic-minded citizens, all of whom were concerned with children's issues. Largely because of their recommendations, in 1912 Congress passed an act creating the Children's Bureau, a federal agency whose purpose was to investigate and report on the problems of children. The creation of the Children's Bureau is an important milestone in the history of child health and welfare.

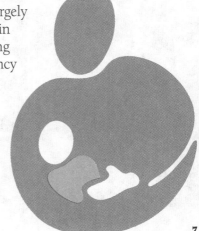

# Child Health in the United States

## Today's Diseases – Today's Docs – Today's Kids

*...and the terrible epidemics ended and the killer diseases disappeared. The children grew strong and healthy, and families rejoiced, and everyone lived happily ever after. The end.*

The "happily-ever-after" ending can be found in children's bedtime stories but rarely in real life. Nevertheless, it's true that the terrible epidemics of diphtheria, measles, and pertussis have ended. And that for the most part, the killer diseases are gone. But there are new threats to our children – substance abuse, eating disorders, teen pregnancy, and more. Yesterday's answers won't always solve today's problems.

New diseases require new approaches. Since many of today's health problems have their roots in emotional and social stresses in the home, school, and community, partnerships between parents, doctors, and schools are increasingly necessary. The new goal for child health care is health promotion – "not just preventing or treating illness or injury, but actively promoting the physical, emotional, mental, and social well-being of children, adolescents, and their families."

*Bright Futures: Guidelines for Health Supervision of Infants, Children, and Adolescents.* 2nd edition.

8

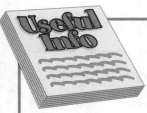

# A Safety Net for Children

The Great Depression of 1929 forced 40 percent of the people of the United States into poverty. The Social Security Act of 1935 created an important safety net for many of those most at risk – the elderly, the disabled, pregnant women, and children.

Title 5 of the Social Security Act created the Maternal and Child Health Services Programs to improve services for the health of mothers and children; children with disabling conditions; homeless, neglected, and delinquent children; and rehabilitation for the physically disabled.

## Medicaid

In 1965, Congress passed Title 19 of the Social Security Act and established Medicaid. Medicaid is a health insurance program for low-income mothers and children, the disabled, and the elderly who meet eligibility requirements. Eligibility varies considerably from state to state. The federal government provides partial funding with states providing matching money. For an eligible child under 21, Medicaid covers all basic medical services, including hospital care, office visits, immunizations, dental care, screening, diagnostic and treatment services.

## Children's Health Insurance Program

In 1997, a major new source of funding for uninsured children was created when Congress passed Title 21 of the Social Security Act. Title 21, the state Children's Health Insurance Program (CHIP), is expected to provide coverage for 10 million uninsured children. For more information, call Hoosier Healthwise at 1-877-KIDS-NOW.

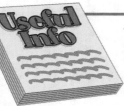

# Riley Hospital for Children

Built to honor the memory of the famous Hoosier poet, James Whitcomb Riley, Riley Hospital for Children opened its doors in October 1924. In the years since, the doctors at Riley have cared for many children with many diseases.

Never were Riley's wards more crowded than during the polio epidemics of 1949 and 1951. The iron lung, one of the earliest "breathing machines," kept paralyzed patients alive until they could breathe on their own.

Today Riley is one of the 10 largest children's hospitals in the nation. The building, the patients, the equipment, and the doctors have all changed, but the reason for Riley remains the same – to bring the best that medicine has to offer to the children and families of Indiana.

## Your Doctor's Office is Your Medical Home

Primary care doctors are your partners for your child's health. They treat ear infections, check growth and development, give "baby shots," and answer middle-of-the-night phone calls.

Emergency rooms only take care of emergencies. "Baby shot clinics" only give "baby shots." Your child's primary care doctor does more. Your doctor provides your child with a medical home.

## A Medical Home Provides...

### Health Care

- Well child care
- Sick child care

- Infants
- Preschoolers
- School-age children
- Teenagers

### Preventive Care

- Immunizations
- Health screenings
- Growth and development checks

- Parenting help
- Behavioral guidance
- Safety precautions

### Coordination of Care

- Physician specialists
- Referrals such as speech and hearing and physical and occupational therapy

- Public health resources
- Health/ Development issues related to child care/ school

### Official Records of Care

- Medical record
- Immunization record

### & Cost-effective Care

Home Sweet Home

# Well Child Care

## The Well Child Visit Schedule

The American Academy of Pediatrics recommends well child visits at the following times:

• Before your baby is born (for first-time parents)

• Before your newborn is discharged from the hospital. If your baby is discharged before two full days of life, your baby should be seen again within 48 and 72 hours.

• During the first year of life – a visit at about 2-4 weeks of age and at 2, 4, 6, 9, and 12 months of age

• During the second year of life – visits at 15, 18, and 24 months of age

• In early childhood – yearly visits from 2-5 years of age

• During early school years – visits at 6, 8, and 10 years of age

• In adolescence and early adulthood – yearly visits from 11-21 years of age

## The Well Child Visit

Well child visits are more important than you might imagine. In addition to providing you and your child with the perfect opportunity to get to know the doctor (and the doctor to get to know the two of you), they allow your doctor to evaluate your child's general health, growth, and development.

When children are sick, they don't feel like showing the doctor how well they walk or talk. They don't relate very well either, so their social skills cannot be evaluated. A well child visit requires a well child. A 6-month-old's appointment for an ear infection can't be used for the 6-month well child visit.

# The Well Child History

At each well child visit, the doctor will ask about:
- History of any illnesses since the last visit
- Daily routine – eating, sleeping, etc.
- Family relationships/friends
- Developmental milestones/puberty
- Child care arrangements
- School
- Any other concerns

When your child is a baby, the doctor takes the history while you hold your child. By age 4 or 5, your child will probably feel comfortable sitting on the exam table during the history. By school age, the doctor spends part of the time talking directly with your child. Once your child becomes a teenager, the doctor will talk with and examine your child without you in the room.

# The Well Child Physical Examination

Each well child visit includes a height and weight check before the exam. In the first 2 years of life, your baby's head size is also measured.

## Height

In the first months of life, length is measured with your child lying down with legs stretched straight. When your child is older (approximately age 2), height is measured while your child is standing. Many times the first height measured on a child is less than the last recorded length. Your child didn't shrink. It's just the difference in the way the height (standing) and length (lying down) are measured.

## Weight

Unlike height, your child's weight changes from day to day and from morning to night. In the first few months of life, small differences may seem very important.

Don't be surprised if your doctor's scale weighs your child heavier or lighter than your scale at home. Remember, your doctor follows your child's weight pattern, which is much more accurate than a single weight.

# Well Child Care

## Head Size

The head grows faster in the first two years than any other time in life. Both your baby's head size and the rate at which your baby's head is growing are important. These measurements help your doctor determine if your child's skull and brain are developing normally.

## Growth

At each visit, your child's height, weight, and head size (in the first two years) are compared to normal values for children of the same age and sex. Your child's measurements are plotted on growth charts from the National Center for Health Statistics like the charts on page 47 of the *Growth and Development* section.

Your child's growth tells your doctor about your child's general health and nutrition. Each child grows differently. Steady

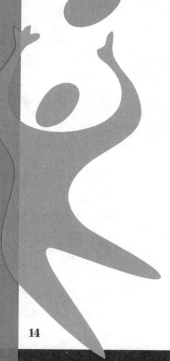

growth is important. A short child who grows steadily is not a worry. A child who stops growing or who loses weight is a worry. By following the growth pattern over a number of months, the normal spurts and slow periods of growth even out.

## General Appearance

Your doctor begins the exam by taking a careful look at your child, checking for a healthy appearance or any signs of health problems. The order of the physical exam changes with the age of the child. With a young child, the doctor usually starts with the parts of the exam requiring cooperation such as listening to the heart and lungs. As the child becomes older, the doctor starts by taking the blood pressure and the examination proceeds head to toe.

# Blood Pressure

Doctors usually begin taking yearly blood pressure measurements at the 3-year well child visit. Normal values for blood pressure change with age and are closely related to height and weight. Normal blood pressure values for children are lower than normal blood pressure values for adults. A normal blood pressure is less than: 105/60 for a 3-year-old; 115/75 for a 10-year-old; and 127/79 for a 15-year-old. (Adult values are considered normal if they are less than 130/85.) Coughing, crying, struggling or anxiety can significantly increase the blood pressure in young children. Children can have high blood pressure for a number of reasons, but frequently it's due to a kidney problem.

## Head

When examining a child under 2, the physician checks the "soft spots" of the skull. Soft spots, or fontanels, are areas where the skull bones have not yet grown together to form a bony, protective shell over the brain.

There are two fontanels that may be open at birth. The fontanel on the back of the head, which is triangular, may be closed at birth, but if not, it closes in the first 4 months of life. The fontanel on the top of the head, which is diamond-shaped, closes by 2 years of age. The closure occurs as the edges of the bones surrounding the fontanel add new bone until the fontanel is finally filled in.

In addition to measuring your child's head size, your doctor checks the shape of your child's head. Young babies who lie with their heads in one position too long can have flattening of that part of the skull.

## Ears

Your doctor checks your child's ears for signs of infection or fluid behind the ear drum. Ear infections are common in young children. Not all children complain of earaches. Untreated ear infections cause problems with speech and hearing. Your doctor checks to make sure a "silent" ear infection is not missed.

If you have any concerns about your child's hearing, be sure to bring them up with your doctor. Children with normal hearing at birth can develop hearing problems because of ear infections or exposure to very loud noises. Parents are frequently the first to notice a hearing problem.

# Well Child Care

## Ears (continued)

Don't be concerned about ear wax and don't use a cotton swab to clean your child's ears because the ear canal is easily injured. If the doctor can't see the ear drum because of ear wax, he or she will take care of the problem very carefully.

## Eyes

Your doctor uses a lighted instrument called an ophthalmoscope to look through the pupil into the back of the eye. The doctor is looking for problems inside the eye like a cataract or a tumor.

The doctor also checks your child's eyes for problems that can be seen from the outside like excessive tearing or eyes that don't move together.

Beginning at age 3, the doctor will probably check your child's vision. If you have a family history of vision problems, particularly of hereditary eye disease, be sure to tell your doctor. Your child will be referred to an ophthalmologist if your doctor suspects problems.

## Nose, Throat, and Mouth

The doctor checks your child's nose for signs of allergy or chronic infection. Your doctor also checks the back of your child's throat for enlarged tonsils or signs of infection.

When examining the mouth, he or she looks at the condition of the teeth and gums. Your doctor's examination of your child's teeth does not substitute for a visit to the dentist. Children should begin regular dental check-ups between ages 2 and 3.

## Neck

Your doctor checks several things with the neck exam. He or she checks to make sure your child's head moves easily from side to side and up and down. The doctor feels the neck for "lumps and bumps" – an enlarged thyroid gland or swollen lymph nodes. Swollen lymph nodes in the back of the neck suggest an infection of the scalp. Swollen lymph nodes in the front of the neck suggest an infection of the tonsils. Swollen lymph nodes behind the ear suggest an ear infection.

## Chest and Lungs

Your doctor will look, listen, and feel during the chest and lung exam. Your doctor observes the rate of breathing, deep or shallow breathing, and easy or labored breathing. The stethoscope is used to listen for normal or abnormal breathing sounds.

## Heart

Your doctor can feel the force of your child's heart beating by feeling the chest wall over the heart. The stethoscope is used to listen for normal or abnormal sounds. Many children have heart murmurs, however, not all of these indicate a problem. If your doctor mentions a murmur, don't be alarmed. If it is serious, your child will be referred to a pediatric heart specialist for further evaluation.

## Abdomen

By gently pressing down on the abdominal wall, your doctor learns if your child's spleen and liver are normal size or enlarged. By pressing deeper, your doctor checks kidney size. Your doctor also checks for any "lumps or bumps" or tenderness in the abdomen.

Using a stethoscope, your doctor can hear the sounds of fluid or food moving through the bowel, which means the intestines are working normally.

The examination of the abdomen can be uncomfortable for ticklish preschoolers and school-age children who frequently start to giggle when the doctor's hand comes close to the child's tummy. It's important for the tummy muscles to be relaxed when your doctor checks for abnormalities. Very likely, your doctor will try to distract your child during the exam. That sometimes helps with the "giggles."

## Genitals

The doctor routinely checks the genitals for rashes and other signs of infection. With both girls and boys, the doctor uses the genital exam to look for signs of sexual maturation. When examining boys, the doctor checks to make sure the testes have descended into the scrotum and that there are no abnormal masses.

## Nervous System

When your child's reflexes are checked, the doctor is looking for problems with the nervous system. Simple tests of coordination and muscle strength combined with the developmental assessment are also used to look for diseases of the nervous system.

## Skeletal System

Your doctor checks for different skeletal problems at different ages. At the early well child visits, your doctor checks to make sure your child does not have a problem with abnormal hip joints. It is important to treat hip problems early to avoid the need for surgery. Your doctor also checks your baby's legs and feet. The baby's cramped position during pregnancy can cause the legs to appear bowed and may cause incurving of the feet. Such problems are temporary and will be outgrown.

Sports injuries are the most frequent cause of bone and joint problems of older children. The next most common skeletal problem your doctor checks for is scoliosis or "S" curving of the back. Frequently, schools screen for scoliosis, and parents are asked to have a child with a positive screening test further evaluated. Scoliosis can be progressive and needs to be diagnosed early so it can be treated. It is more common in girls than in boys.

## Skin

At each visit, the doctor will examine your child's skin for rashes, birthmarks, bruising, infection, or changes in moles. The skin may provide the first clue of an illness such as leukemia or problems with the nervous system.

In the teen years, acne will be a primary concern – more for your teenager than for the doctor. There are lots of things to do to make sure your child doesn't end up with permanent scarring from untreated acne. Be sure to ask your doctor for help or for referral to a dermatologist.

## Development

Just as your doctor watches over your child's growth, he or she follows your child's development. Children are constantly changing, adding new skills in every area: *social development*, which includes how your child interacts with you and others; *language development*, which includes everything from cooing to talking in sentences; *gross motor skills*, which include large muscle movements involving the arms and legs like throwing a ball or walking; and *fine motor skills*, which include using fingers and hands for drawing or coloring. By following your child's development over time, your doctor is able to identify possible problems with development and refer your child for early intervention.

# Well Child Care

## Talking with the Doctor

If the best part of the well child visit is watching your child show off new developmental skills, the second best part is having the opportunity to talk about your child with an expert one-on-one! You can check out an armload of books from the library, log on to an up-to-the-minute child care Web site, or spend hours trading stories with other parents. However, not one of these valuable resources matches the individualized support and professional expertise available to you at each well child visit. Take advantage of this golden opportunity. Go prepared. Check out the list below for age-appropriate discussion topics.

### 1 month
Crying
Colic
Thumb sucking
Pacifiers
Sleep
Temperament

### 2 months
Child care
Returning to work

### 4 months
Talking to your baby
Teething
Bedtime routine
Age-appropriate toys
Reading to your baby

### 6 months
Talking to your baby
Daily routine
Self-comfort
Transitional object
(stuffed animal)

### 9 months
Talking to your baby
Safe exploration
Simple rules like
"don't touch"
Transitional object
Bedtime routine

### 1 year
Behavior
Language development
Safe play
Consistent rules
Hitting, biting
Self-quieting

### 15 months
Curiosity
Power struggles
Negative behavior

### 18 months
Appropriate language
Power struggles
Praising positive
behavior
Night waking, night
fears, nightmares
Sharing

### 2 years
Praising positive
behavior
Appropriate language
Parallel play
Limits and structure
Toilet training

## 3 years

Praising positive behavior
Preschool readiness
Reading
Physical activity
Fears
Genital exploration/ masturbation

## 4 years

Praising positive behavior
School readiness
Family chores

## 5 years

Health habits
TV limits
Bedtime 7-8 p.m.
Personal care and hygiene
Hand washing

## 6 years

Team sports
Family chores
Teaching child right and wrong
Self-control
Impulse control
Managing anger
Child's friends
School performance
Discipline

## 8 years

Healthy habits
Tobacco, alcohol, drug education
Education about pubertal changes
Peer relationships
Reading

## 10 years

Bedtime 8-9 p.m.
Hobbies
Homework spot
Acceptance of diversity
Opportunities for success
Education about pubertal changes

## 11-14 years

Sleep
TV and computer limits
Time management
Family time
Team sports
Family rules
Sexuality issues, sex identification, abstinence, protected sex, sexually-transmitted diseases (STDs)
Substance abuse, alcohol, tobacco

## 15-17 years

Stress
Feelings
Challenges
School work
Life plans
Safe driving
New skills like life saving, peer mentoring
Sexuality issues, STDs, abstinence
Substance abuse, alcohol, tobacco

# Dental Care

## Dental Facts

- Baby bottle tooth decay is the most common cause of tooth decay in a child younger than 3 years.

- The chewing surfaces of back teeth are the most likely to decay. Sixty-six percent of cavities occur in the back teeth.

- The ideal time for placement of braces is 8-14 years of age because the head and mouth are still growing and teeth can be more easily straightened. Usually braces are worn for 18-30 months, and then a retainer is worn for a few months to two years.

### Health Alert — Protect Your Child's Teeth

Children playing contact sports should wear a mouth guard. A mouth guard may be purchased at any sporting goods store.

If your child has front teeth that protrude, you should discuss the problem with your dentist. The risk of broken teeth is far greater if your child has protruding front teeth.

A child with a neuromuscular disorder or frequent seizures should wear a helmet and mouth guard to protect the head and face during falls.

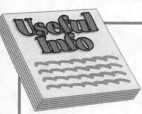

# Good News for Parents

Before the age of 3 years, it is unlikely that using a pacifier or thumb or finger sucking will cause any permanent harm to your baby's teeth or smile. The children most likely to have significant dental problems use a pacifier (or suck their thumb or finger) frequently for long periods of time and continue the habit after 3 years of age. Thumb or finger sucking is the hardest habit to break – 20 percent of children continue the habit after age 5.

# Call Your Dentist

### If a baby tooth is knocked out

If a baby tooth is knocked out, there is no way to "save" the tooth. If the gum is bleeding, cover your finger with gauze and press down on the bleeding area. Call your dentist to determine if he or she feels it is necessary to fit your child with a "spacer." A "spacer" takes the place of the baby tooth and holds the place for the permanent tooth until it comes in.

### If a permanent tooth is knocked out

Rinse (but do not scrub) the tooth, holding it by its crown. Do not touch the roots. It is wise to plug the drain before you begin rinsing. Insert the tooth into the socket with gentle pressure. Replace the tooth quickly, within 20 minutes if possible. It is uncommon for the tooth to survive if replacement is delayed longer than two hours. Take your child to the dentist immediately so that the tooth can be immobilized.

If you are unable to replace the tooth, take your child and the tooth to the dentist. Transport the tooth in milk.

*"All I want for Christmas is my two front teeth"*

# Dental Care

## Clean Teeth are Healthy Teeth

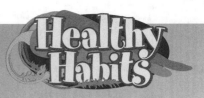

- Put only water in your baby's naptime or bedtime bottle.
- Wipe your baby's gums with a clean, damp cloth after each feeding.
- Start brushing your baby's teeth as soon as the first tooth appears.
- Nonfluoride toothpaste in small amounts should be used beginning at 12 months of age.
- Schedule your child's first dental visit before the age of 3 years.
- By age 4-5 years, children are usually able to brush their own teeth. However, to ensure thorough cleaning, their toothbrushing should be supervised until age 7 years.
- Children should use a pea-sized amount of fluoride toothpaste. Fluoride toothpaste should not be used until the child is old enough to spit out the extra toothpaste and rinse with water after brushing.
- Once all the baby teeth have come in, you should floss your child's teeth. Children can usually floss alone after age 8, although you may need to supervise them.

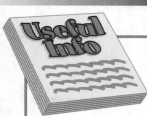

# Tooth Eruption Charts

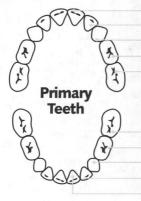

**Primary Teeth**

| Upper Teeth | Erupt | Shed |
|---|---|---|
| Central incisor | 8-12 mos. | 6-7 yrs. |
| Lateral incisor | 9-13 mos. | 7-8 yrs. |
| Canine (cuspid) | 16-22 mos. | 10-12 yrs. |
| First molar | 13-19 mos. | 9-11 yrs. |
| Second molar | 25-33 mos. | 10-12 yrs. |

| Lower Teeth | Erupt | Shed |
|---|---|---|
| Second molar | 23-31 mos. | 10-12 yrs. |
| First molar | 14-18 mos. | 9-11 yrs. |
| Canine (cuspid) | 17-23 mos. | 9-12 yrs. |
| Lateral incisor | 10-16 mos. | 7-8 yrs. |
| Central incisor | 6-10 mos. | 6-7 yrs. |

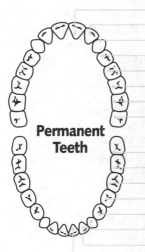

**Permanent Teeth**

| Upper Teeth | Erupt |
|---|---|
| Central incisor | 7-8 yrs. |
| Lateral incisor | 8-9 yrs. |
| Canine (cuspid) | 11-12 yrs. |
| First premolar (first bicuspid) | 10-11 yrs. |
| Second premolar (second bicuspid) | 10-12 yrs. |
| First molar | 6-7 yrs. |
| Second molar | 12-13 yrs. |
| Third molar (wisdom tooth) | 17-21 yrs. |

| Lower Teeth | Erupt |
|---|---|
| Third molar (wisdom tooth) | 17-21 yrs. |
| Second molar | 11-13 yrs. |
| First molar | 6-7 yrs. |
| Second premolar (second bicuspid) | 11-12 yrs. |
| First premolar (first bicuspid) | 10-12 yrs. |
| Canine (cuspid) | 9-10 yrs. |
| Lateral incisor | 7-8 yrs. |
| Central incisor | 6-7 yrs. |

Source: American Dental Association

# Eye Care

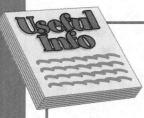

## Eye Facts

- Babies look like they have big eyes at birth because they do. The eye of the newborn is about 65 percent the size of the adult eye.

- Babies may not have tears when they cry until they are between 1 and 3 months old.

- Although babies can see at birth and especially enjoy looking at faces, they do not see as well as adults until 1 year of age.

- Early in life, babies see strong, bright colors the best. They are also attracted to bold patterns in black and white. Pale pinks and blues, which are traditionally considered baby colors, probably aren't even noticed by babies.

- At age 3-4 months, your baby's vision has developed so that he or she can see small objects. Some babies start to have color vision at this age.

- By 4 months of age, your child will have developed 3D (three dimensional) vision.

- Children who are nearsighted have difficulty seeing objects that are far away. Nearsightedness is the most common vision problem in young children. Nearsightedness is inherited and is usually not diagnosed until after 3-4 years of age. Nearsightedness is not caused by reading too much or by reading in dim light.

- Children who are farsighted must focus a bit harder to see objects up close but rarely need glasses unless the condition is severe.

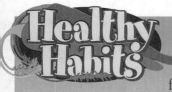

## Here's Looking at You, Kid

Your child's eyes should be examined at the following times:

*Newborn:* Your doctor checks your baby's eyes during the newborn physical examination. Be certain to tell your doctor if you have a family history of eye disease, including loss of vision in childhood or the need to wear thick glasses at an early age.

If your newborn has an obvious eye problem, is premature, or has multiple medical problems, your doctor will ask an ophthalmologist to check your baby's eyes.

*Age 6 months:* Your doctor will check your baby's eyes to be sure they are moving together. Be sure to mention habitual head tilting or watery eyes.

*Age 3-4 years:* Your doctor will check your child's vision at the well child visit. Your child does not have to be able to read. Doctors can use pictures or a simple chart to test visual acuity.

*Age 5 years:* Your child's vision should be rechecked before school entry and at the routine well child visits.

## Child Rearing Myth

Some people think that if a child uses a computer for long periods of time, it will damage his or her eyes.

## Child Rearing Fact

Using a computer for long periods of time does not cause eye damage. However, whenever your child does close work, he or she blinks less and the eyes become dry. This dryness may lead to the sensation of eye strain and tired eyes. It's a good habit to teach your child to look up from the computer (or from a book or other close activity) and focus on a distant object at least every 15 or 20 minutes.

# Eye Care

## Ask Your Doctor

The first few years of life are critical to the development of normal vision. Normal vision depends on normal function of the eye and the area of the brain devoted to vision. The best chance for normal vision exists when eye diseases or vision problems are diagnosed before the fifth year of life. Parents are frequently the first to notice an eye problem. Call your doctor if you notice any of the following…

*At 2-3 months:*

- Your baby is unable to "look you in the eye," does not have steady eye contact, or seems unable to see.

- Your baby's eyes do not move together most of the time, or one eye frequently turns out or in. (All babies cross their eyes occasionally in the first few months.)

*At older than 3 months:*

- Your baby is unable to follow an object even if it is brightly colored and moves slowly in front of the baby's face.

*At any age:*

- The pupils of your child's eyes are of unequal size.

- Your child holds objects close in order to see them.

- Your child's eyes flutter from side to side or up and down.

- Your child rubs his or her eyes frequently.

- Your child squints to see or turns his or her head to one side.

- Your child has redness in either eye that persists for several days.

- Your child has redness, swelling, crusting, or discharge affecting one or both eyes and lasting more than 24 hours.

- Your child's eyes appear to be crossed, turned out, or not focusing together.

- One or both of your child's eyelids appear to droop.

- One or both of your child's eyes appear to bulge.

- Your child has an eye injury.

Most likely, you have never seen a child with diphtheria or heard the "whoop" of whooping cough (pertussis). While these diseases have almost disappeared because of immunizations, they are still killing children in other countries. It's important for all parents to remember that children can still be exposed to these diseases by simply flying in an airplane or by visiting a foreign country.

# Hepatitis B

Hepatitis B is a serious liver disease caused by a virus. The hepatitis B virus is spread by contact with blood or other body fluids of an infected person. Hepatitis B can enter the blood stream, attack the liver, and cause severe illness – even death.

Infants and children who become infected with the hepatitis B virus are at the highest risk of developing lifelong infection, which often leads to death from liver disease and liver cancer. Approximately 25 percent of children who become infected with lifelong hepatitis B virus die of related liver disease as adults.

Source: Centers for Disease Control & Prevention

# Diphtheria
## Given as Diphtheria, Tetanus, Acellular Pertussis – DTaP

Diphtheria is a serious disease caused by poison produced from the bacteria. It frequently causes heart and nerve problems. The death rate is 5 percent to 10 percent, with higher rates (up to 20 percent) in the very young.

In the 1920s, diphtheria was a major cause of illness and death for children in the United States. Although diphtheria is rare in the United States, it is still a threat. Diphtheria is common in other parts of the world.

Source: Centers for Disease Control & Prevention

# Immunizations

## Pertussis
### Given as Diphtheria, Tetanus, Acellular Pertussis – DTaP

Pertussis (whooping cough) is most severe during the first year of life. Even in older children, it can cause prolonged coughing spells that last for many weeks. These spells make eating, drinking, and breathing difficult. When the coughing spells cause vomiting, infants lose weight and become dehydrated. Other complications of pertussis include pneumonia, seizures, central nervous system involvement, and rarely death.

Source: Centers for Disease Control & Prevention

## Tetanus
### Given as Diphtheria, Tetanus, Acellular Pertussis – DTaP

Tetanus is a severe, often fatal disease. The bacteria that cause tetanus are widely distributed in soil and street dust, are found in the waste of many animals, and are resistant to heat and germ-killing cleaners.

People who get tetanus suffer from stiffness and spasms of the muscles. The larynx (windpipe) can close, causing breathing difficulties. Muscle spasms can be so severe that they cause bone fractures. Some people go into a coma and die. Approximately 30 percent of people who develop tetanus die.

Source: Centers for Disease Control & Prevention

# Polio
## Given as Inactivated Polio Virus - IPV

The polio virus can cause minor infections that heal after a few days or rapidly progressive, serious infections that are complicated by paralysis, permanent physical disability, and even death. Before the polio vaccine was available in the United States, 13,000 to 20,000 cases of paralytic polio occurred each year. These annual epidemics left thousands of victims – mostly children – in braces, crutches, and wheelchairs for life.

Source: Centers for Disease Control & Prevention

# Pneumococcus

Pneumococcal infections include ear infections, sinusitis, pneumonia, and meningitis. All of these diseases can have serious complications. Pneumococcal disease kills about 40,000 people each year.

Source: Centers for Disease Control & Prevention

# Measles
## Given as Measles, Mumps, Rubella - MMR

Before the measles vaccine was available, nearly everyone in the United States got measles (7-day measles). There were approximately 3-4 million cases each year. As many as 20 percent of people with measles required hospitalization, and almost 10 percent suffered complications such as diarrhea, ear infections, or pneumonia. When the virus infected the brain, permanent damage to brain function occurred.

Measles is one of the most infectious diseases in the world. More than 90 percent of people who are not immune will develop measles if they are exposed to the virus. In 1998, most cases of measles were associated with international visitors or United States residents who were exposed to the measles virus while traveling abroad.

Source: Centers for Disease Control & Prevention

# Immunizations

## Mumps
### Given as Measles, Mumps, Rubella - MMR

Before the mumps vaccine was introduced, mumps was a major cause of deafness in children, occurring in approximately 1 per 20,000 reported cases. Mumps is usually a mild viral disease. However, rare conditions such as swelling of the brain, nerves, and spinal cord can lead to serious side effects such as paralysis and seizures.

Serious side effects of mumps are more common in adults than children. Swelling of the testes is the most common side effect in males past the age of puberty, occurring in up to 20 percent to 50 percent of men who become ill with mumps. An increase in miscarriage has been found among women who develop mumps in the first three months of their pregnancy. If the mumps vaccination were to stop, the number of cases could go back to prevaccine levels of more than 200,000 cases per year.

Source: Centers for Disease Control & Prevention

## Rubella
### Given as Measles, Mumps, Rubella - MMR

While rubella (German measles, 3-day measles) is usually mild in children and adults, up to 90 percent of infants born to mothers who become infected with rubella in the first three months of pregnancy will develop congenital rubella syndrome, resulting in heart defects, cataracts, mental retardation, and deafness.

Source: Centers for Disease Control & Prevention

## Haemophilus Influenzae (Hib)

Before the Hib vaccine became available, Haemophilus influenzae was the most common cause of bacterial meningitis in infants and children, affecting about 16,000 children in the United States each year. One in 20 children with Haemophilus meningitis died. Twenty percent to 30 percent of the survivors were left with permanent brain damage.

Source: Centers for Disease Control & Prevention

# Varicella

Varicella (chickenpox) is always present in the community and is highly contagious. Before licensing of the chickenpox vaccine in 1995, almost every adult in the United States had been infected by the virus. Chickenpox was responsible for an estimated 4 million illnesses, 11,000 hospitalizations, and 100 deaths each year.

Chickenpox is usually mild, but may be severe. Complications such as bacterial infections, loss of fluids (dehydration), pneumonia, and central nervous system involvement can occur. Furthermore, even after the chickenpox infection has healed, the inactivated virus remains in the body and can cause another problem – shingles. Shingles, a painful rash occurring when the inactive virus living in a nerve becomes active, affects about 300,000 people each year. Only people who have had chickenpox can get shingles.

Source: Centers for Disease Control & Prevention

# Vaccination Schedule

| Birth | 2 months | 4 months | 6 months |
|---|---|---|---|
| Hepatitis B #1 | DTaP #1 | Polio (IPV) #2 | DTaP #3 |
| | Polio (IPV) #1 | Hib #2 | Hib #3 |
| | Hib #1 | DTaP #2 | Pneumococcus #3 |
| | Hepatitis B #2 | Pneumococcus #2 | |
| | Pneumococcus #1 | | |

| 12 months | 15 months | 18 months | 4-6 years |
|---|---|---|---|
| MMR #1 | Hib #4 | Polio (IPV) #3 | MMR #2 |
| Varicella | Hepatitis B #3 | DTaP #4 | Polio (IPV) #4 |
| (Chickenpox) | Pneumococcus #4 | | DTaP #5 |

| 11-12 years |
|---|
| Tetanus, Diphtheria booster (Td) |
| The following vaccines should be given if previously recommended doses were missed or given earlier than the recommended age: Hepatitis B, MMR, Varicella (chickenpox). |

Childhood Immunization Schedule – US, Jan-Dec 2001, approved by the Advisory Committee on Immunization Practices, the American Academy of Pediatrics and the American Academy of Family Physicians.

# Sick Child Basics

Why is sickness in a child such a worry? If you become ill, you probably wait four or five days before even thinking of calling your doctor. If your child becomes ill, you have to talk yourself into waiting to make the call to the doctor until you have taken your child's temperature. Most parents – especially first-time parents – call the doctor's office more than necessary. But doctors would rather have you call too often and too early than too late.

Doctors know that it's difficult for parents to tell when a child is seriously ill and that a child can get very sick very quickly.

## Keep it to Yourself

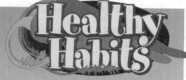

Anyone who cares for your child should know and use these habits to limit the spread of infection:

- Wash hands after changing diapers, going to the bathroom, cleaning up soiled linens or soiled clothing.

- Do not share combs, brushes, or hats.

- Do not share drinking glasses, bottles, or silverware.

- Do not share toothbrushes. Purchase a new toothbrush after your child recovers from an illness. Discard old toothbrush.

- Protect skin in areas of constant moisture and irritation (nose with cold, diaper area with diarrhea) from cracks and sores that may become infected.

- Wash hands after wiping nose or using nose syringe for baby's nose. To prevent the spread of infection from nose to eye, keep hands away from eyes after blowing nose or touching nose.

# How Sick is Sick?

When your child is sick, get into the habit of checking your child's temperature and observing your child closely. Unconsciousness, difficulty breathing or abnormal color (very pale or blue) are obvious signs of serious illness. More subtle signs (listed below) can also help you decide the seriousness of your child's illness.

## Checking for Signs of Serious Illness

### Appearance

**Reassuring Signs:** Your child appears "bright-eyed" and alert.

**Worrisome Signs:** Your child appears sleepy with "dull" eyes and little expression on his or her face.

**Serious-Illness-Likely Signs:** Your child just stares "blankly" and has a "glassy-eyed" look.

### Cry

**Reassuring Signs:** Your child cries in the usual way at the usual things.

**Worrisome Signs:** Your child's cry sound whiny. Your child is difficult to comfort and whimpers off and on.

**Serious-Illness-Likely Signs:** Your child's cry sounds weak. Your child continues to cry or moan even when being comforted.

### Activity Level

**Reassuring Signs:** Your child plays and sleeps normally.

**Worrisome Signs:** Your child is fussy when awake and sleeps more than usual.

**Serious-Illness-Likely Signs:** Your child is hard to awaken and has little or no interest in playing.

### Appetite

**Reassuring Signs:** Your child asks for favorite foods and liquids and eats and drinks the requested foods and liquids.

**Worrisome Signs:** Your child takes liquids or food if offered, but takes only a few sips of liquid or a few bites of food.

**Serious-Illness-Likely Signs:** Your child pushes away or refuses all food and liquids.

# Sick Child Basics

## Checking for Signs of Serious Illness (continued)
### Urination

**Reassuring Signs:** Your child voids (pees) light yellow urine with the usual frequency. A baby should have 6-8 wet diapers a day.

**Worrisome Signs:** Your child voids dark yellow urine less frequently than usual.

**Serious-Illness-Likely Signs:** Your child appears "dry" and his or her eyes appear to have sunk back into the head. Your child has very little saliva (spit) and very little urine.

If all of the signs in all of the areas are "reassuring," feel reassured that for the time being, your child is not seriously ill. However, remember that your child's condition can change, so you'll need to recheck signs on a regular basis. If your child has one or two "worrisome" signs, it's a good idea to report these to your doctor's office and ask for advice. If your child has three or more "worrisome" signs, call the doctor's office immediately to report your observations and to request an appointment for your child. When "serious-illness-likely" signs are present, it is important to act quickly to make arrangements with your doctor to have your child examined without delay.

# Making the Call

When you make the call to your doctor, begin with a report of your child's temperature. Tell the doctor your child's temperature, how it was taken, and the time and amount of the most recent fever medicine. Next, briefly go over when your child became ill, your child's symptoms, and any signs that are "worrisome" or that "serious illness is likely." Have pen and paper ready to write down the doctor's instructions. Don't be afraid to ask questions or have information repeated.

# When Your Baby is Sick

In the first 3 months of life, it's particularly important to call the doctor if your baby is sick. Call your doctor immediately for a temperature higher than 100.4° F. **DO NOT USE ASPIRIN TO BRING THE FEVER DOWN.** If other symptoms such as excessive fussiness, excessive sleepiness, refusal to eat, and/or coughing are present, seek care immediately.

# The All-Too-Common Cold

In the first 3-4 years of life, children catch an average of 6-8 colds a year. The average cold lasts three weeks. If you add up the time that your child is catching a cold, sick with a cold, and getting over a cold, almost half of the year is "cold season."

Until a child is old enough to blow his or her nose, mucus from the nose drains into the back of the throat and is swallowed into the stomach. By clearing the mucus with a nose syringe, you can make your baby more comfortable. The use of saline nose drops makes the mucus easier to remove. Saline nose drops can be purchased over the counter (without a doctor's prescription). Babies with colds sleep better if placed in a semi-sitting position in a pumpkin seat rather than flat on their backs because they are less likely to be bothered by draining mucus.

# Sick Child Basics

## Call Your Doctor
### Infectious disease alert

*Your child may need protection*

If your child is exposed to hepatitis or meningitis, call your doctor. Provide the doctor with the name and phone number of the individual who notified you so the doctor can follow up, if necessary.

## Over-the-Counter Medications

**Health Alert**

*Do not use over-the-counter (OTC) medicines without checking with your doctor.*

There are lots of over-the-counter medicines that adults use that should not be used for children. **It's not just a matter of adjusting the dosage.** Many drugs can cause harmful side effects in children. Although the pharmacist is a wonderful source of information about prescriptions and over-the-counter medications, you should not substitute his or her advice for your doctor's OK.

Take the following over-the-counter medication list to your child's next well child visit. Ask your doctor about using these medications. Write down the name and the dosage of any drug your doctor OKs. Also write down any warnings.

- Cold preparations including all combination medications for a cough, fever, runny nose
- Sleep medications
- Medications to dry up a stuffy nose
- Medication for vomiting
- Medication to stop diarrhea
- Antihistamines or decongestants

# When to Keep Your Child Home

The American Academy of Pediatrics recommends that your child be kept home from child care or school if any of the following conditions exist…

- A child with any signs of severe illness, including fever, irritability, difficulty breathing, crying that does not stop with the usual comforting, or extreme sleepiness should not be sent to child care or school.

- A child with diarrhea or stools that contain blood or mucus should not attend child care or school.

- A child who vomits two or more times in 24 hours should not attend child care or school, unless a physician feels the cause of vomiting is not an infectious disease and the child is in no danger of becoming dehydrated.

- A child with mouth sores and drooling should not attend child care or school, unless a physician or the local health department authority does not feel the condition is infectious.

- A child with fever or rash or a change in behavior should not attend school or child care, unless a physician has determined that the problem is not caused by an infectious disease.

- A child with diarrhea caused by E-coli 0157:H7 or shigella that has been diagnosed by a physician should not attend child care or school. The child may not return to day care or school until two stool cultures (collected 24 hours apart) are negative for the organisms and the child no longer has diarrhea. For shigella, the child may return if treated with an appropriate antibiotic for five days and if the child no longer has diarrhea.

- A child with conjunctivitis or "pinkeye" may not attend day care or school without being examined, treated, and approved for readmission by a physician.

- A child with impetigo may not attend school or day care until 24 hours after beginning antibiotic treatment and until the child no longer has a fever. Be sure to cover any lesions.

- A child with strep throat may not attend school or day care until 24 hours after beginning antibiotic treatment.

# Sick Child Basics

## When to Keep Your Child Home (continued)

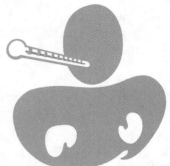

- A child with head lice may not attend day care or school until the first treatment has been given.

- A child with scabies may not attend day care or school until after treatment has been completed.

- A child with chickenpox must remain out of day care or school until all lesions are dried and crusted, which is usually after about six days.

- A child with pertussis (whooping cough) must remain out of school or day care until five days of antibiotic treatment have been completed. (Treatment is to continue for a total of 14 days.)

- A child with mumps may not return to school or day care until nine days after the swelling begins.

- A child with measles must remain out of school or child care until four days after the rash begins.

- A child with hepatitis A must remain out of school or child care until one week after the child develops jaundice (yellow skin color) or becomes ill.

- A child with tuberculosis must remain out of school or child care until the child's physician or local health department authority feels the child's condition is no longer infectious.

- A child with an illness that prevents the child from feeling well enough to participate in the usual activities and routines should not be sent to school or child care.

*For child care only: A child whose illness requires more care than the child care staff can provide without putting the health and safety of other children at risk should not be sent to child care.*

# Resources

## Organizations

*American Academy of Pediatrics*
141 Northwest Point Boulevard
P.O. Box 747
Elk Grove Village, Illinois 60009-0747
800-433-9016 (phone)
847-228-1281 (fax)
www.aap.org

*American Dental Association*
Department of Public Information and Education
211 East Chicago Avenue
Chicago, Illinois 60611
800-621-8099 (phone)
www.ada.org

*Centers for Disease Control and Prevention*
1600 Clifton Road
Atlanta, Georgia 30333
404-639-3311 (phone)
www.cdc.gov

*National Immunization Program*
*Centers for Disease Control and Prevention*
1600 Clifton Road, MSE-34
Atlanta, Georgia 30333
800-232-2522 (immunization hotline)
www.cdc.gov/nip/

*Indiana State Department of Health*
2 North Meridian Street
Indianapolis, Indiana 46204
317-233-1325 (phone)
www.state.in.us/isdh/

# Resources

*Riley Hospital for Children*
702 Barnhill Drive
Indianapolis, Indiana 46202-5200
317-274-5000
www.rileyhospital.org

*Riley Hospital Community Education Department*
Riley Hospital for Children
575 West Drive, Room 008
Indianapolis, Indiana 46202-5272
317-274-2964 (phone)
317-274-3221 (fax)
www.rileyforkids.org
Provides educational resources on child health, safety and advocacy appropriate for children, parents, and professionals.

*United States Food and Drug Administration*
5600 Fishers Lane
Rockville, Maryland 20857
888-INFO-FDA (888-463-6332)
www.fda.gov

# Recommended Books

*Caring for Your Baby and Young Child: Birth to Age 5*
American Academy of Pediatrics, 1991, Bantam Books.

*Caring for Your School-Age Child: Ages 5-12*
American Academy of Pediatrics, 1995, Bantam Books.

*Caring for Your Adolescent: Ages 12-21*
American Academy of Pediatrics, 1991, Bantam Books.

*Guide to Your Child's Symptoms*
American Academy of Pediatrics, 1997, Bantam Books.

# Web Sites for Parents and Kids

*Beansprout*
www.beansprout.net/family/main.asp

*Food and Drug Administration Kids Page*
www.fda.gov/oc/opacom/kids/default.htm

*Kids Health (Parents, Teens, and Kids)*
www.kidshealth.org

*Riley Hospital Community Education Department*
www.rileyforkids.org

# Growth and Development
## Section Two

## In this Section:

- Physical Growth
- Major Milestones
- Emotional Health
- Brain Facts
- Parents, Kids and Books
- And Much More...

The years between birth announcements and graduation invitations are filled with joys, worries, proud celebrations, and sleepless nights – lots of sleepless nights! All along the way, you'll have more questions than answers.

Browse through the pages in this section for insights on every age and stage. While you're at it, check out the great resources at the end of the section and lots of other useful information and hard-to-find facts about growth and development.

# Tracking Your Child's Growth

Within minutes of your baby's birth, your baby is weighed and measured – weight, length, and head size. The measurements are recorded on the standardized growth chart. Each time your child is seen for a well child visit, weight, length, and head size (for the appropriate age) are measured and charted on the same growth record. (After age 2, the head size is no longer routinely measured.)

# All about Growth Records

## The Growth Chart

Healthy children grow at very different rates. The standard growth chart uses "percentile lines" to display the wide range of normal measurements for different ages.

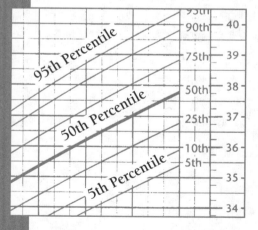

## Comparing Size to Age

**95th percentile** – Large, only 4 of every 100 children are larger at this age.

**50th percentile** – Right in the middle in size at this age.

**5th percentile** – Small, only 4 of every 100 children are smaller at this age.

## The growth chart allows your child's doctor to:

- Track your child's growth – height, weight, and head size – over time.

- Compare your child's growth with the growth of other children of the same sex and age.

# Sample Growth Chart for Length

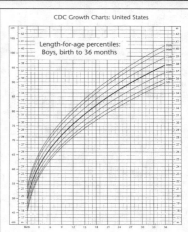

AGE (months)

# Sample Growth Chart for Weight

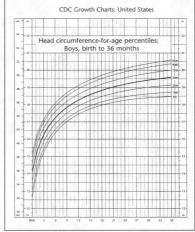

AGE (months)

# Sample Growth Chart for Head Size

AGE (months)

47

## Physical Growth
### How Big is Baby?

A full-term baby born after nine months (38-42 weeks) of pregnancy:

- weighs an average of 7-1/2 pounds

- is an average of 20 inches long

- measures an average head size of almost 14 inches when the tape measure is placed just above the ears and goes around the forehead to the largest part of the back of the head.

Babies have much bigger heads in relation to their bodies than older children or adults. A newborn's head makes up 1/4 of body length. In adults, the head makes up 1/8 of total height.

### Useful Info

## Cold Costs Calories

When you get cold, you shiver and produce body heat by muscle activity. Babies cannot shiver. Instead, they use a special kind of fat to make heat chemically.

The calories used to make chemical heat are calories the baby should be using for growth or normal activity. Putting a warm hat on your baby on a cold day saves "go-and-grow" calories.

# Brain Fact

In the 1990s, research on the developing brain made headlines and nightly news. The Decade of the Brain, as Congress officially proclaimed the 1990s, had important lessons for parents. These are discussed in "Brain Facts" throughout the *Growth and Development* section.

Babies are born with 100 billion nerve cells – almost all of the nerve cells the brain will ever have. Before birth, nerve cells are formed at 250,000 cells per minute.

# Dental Development
## Invisible Teeth

Your baby's teeth begin to form in the third month of pregnancy. The tooth buds, which will develop into the 20 "baby" or primary teeth, form first. Next, the permanent teeth begin to form, and the primary teeth begin to calcify. This process continues throughout the nine months of pregnancy.

When a newborn comes into the world, hidden beneath the gums lies a full set of primary teeth in the process of being calcified, as well as some of the 32 permanent teeth well on their way in the process of development.

# Growth Facts

The best predictor of adult height is the family history – the height of the mother and father. Birth size reflects intrauterine nutrition and factors associated with the pregnancy. By the end of the 2nd year, the child's height reflects the genetic heritage.

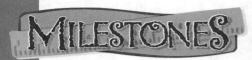

## Making Sense of the World

The five senses – sight, smell, taste, hearing, and touch – are mostly developed at birth. Your baby begins using his or her senses immediately to make sense of what is going on in the world.

*Sight:* Although newborns have blurry vision, they can focus fairly well on objects at about 8 to 14 inches – the distance from your baby's face to your face when you are holding your baby in your arms.

*Smell:* Newborns have a very well-developed sense of smell that makes them very choosy about their favorite scent. In the first days of life, a newborn can recognize his or her mother's natural scent and likes it best of all.

*Taste:* Newborns also have a well-developed sense of taste. They like sweet tastes. Nursing infants sometimes refuse to nurse when they taste garlic or heavy spices in mom's breast milk.

*Hearing:* Babies can hear while they are still inside the womb. At birth, they can recognize their mother's voice – because they have heard it for several months.

*Touch:* Gentle touch is a true pleasure for your newborn. It stimulates physical development while relieving stress. Fussy babies are sometimes calmed by a "baby massage" – some baby lotion warmed in your hands and gently applied to baby's arms, legs, and back.

# Brain Fact

Thanks to new imaging technology, scientists are actually able to watch the brain at work. Research confirms that the most active areas in the newborn's brain are the areas concerned with sight, smell, taste, sound, and touch.

These areas "register" the world as the baby senses it. Then the signals are sent on to memory or emotion. In this way, the newborn connects the sight and smell of mom and dad with the pleasant memory of comfort and gentle handling.

Useful Info

## All Tucked In

In the first month of life, "swaddling" soothes some babies. Bundling the baby so that the arms and legs are tucked up against the body in a flexed position recreates the natural position of babies inside the mother's womb.

Babies who are overstimulated by their own uncontrolled arm and leg movements frequently calm down and become more alert with swaddling. If your baby protests or looks or feels warm when swaddled, unwrap your baby immediately.

# Play Activities
## Baby See, Baby Do

*How?* Hold your baby directly in front of you with your faces about 9 inches apart. Stick out your tongue. Your baby may imitate you. Try opening your mouth.

*Why?* Babies love to look at faces. Many times they will imitate what they see.

## Emotional Development
### Getting Off to the Right Start

- You begin to bond to your baby even before the baby is born. After your baby's birth, your feelings deepen and grow as you get to know your baby, understand your baby's needs, and find pleasure in meeting those needs. You bring pleasure to your baby just as your baby brings pleasure to you. This bond between you, called attachment, provides the essential building block for a lifetime of healthy relationships.

- Dads who "step right up" to the crib and get involved with the care and comforting of their newborns have the best "batting averages" for knowing how to calm babies (and mothers) in distress. Practice makes perfect.

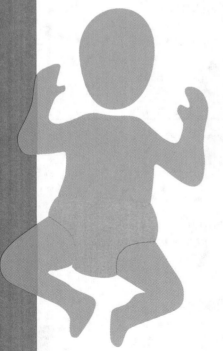

- "Hey, folks, I need a break." When your baby uses body language such as turning or looking away or arching backwards while being held or talked to, your baby may be asking for a little space. Whimpers, cries or fussing when someone is "up close" may be saying the same thing.

# Postpartum Depression

*If you find yourself depressed after your baby is born, especially if your sadness lasts for more than a few days, talk with your partner, your family, or friends. Be frank about your need for help. The doctor who delivered your baby is an excellent resource for professional help.*

Mothers who are sad have few smiles for their babies and may resent caregiving demands. Babies may be stressed, frustrated, or confused by their mother's unresponsiveness. Both mother and baby need help.

# Child Rearing Myth

If you go to your baby every time he or she cries, you will "spoil" your baby.

# Child Rearing Fact

Responding to crying does not spoil babies. Babies are helpless, and they have little they can do to calm themselves. Crying is their wordless way of asking for help. By always responding to your baby's cry for help, you make your baby feel secure and help your child develop a sense of trust. The two most important gifts you give your baby are a sense of trust and the feeling of being safe.

# Brain Fact

Your baby's early experiences are so important that they change the structure of your baby's brain and will have a lifelong effect on his or her ability to learn and on emotional make-up.

## Handwashing

**Healthy Habits**

*To protect your baby, be sure everyone caring for your baby knows this...*

Babies need to be protected from the germs that cause infection. Because a newborn's defense system is immature, even minor skin infections can spread through the body and become life threatening. Prevention is the answer and handwashing is the best prevention.

The most effective way to wash your hands is to scrub them vigorously with warm soapy water for at least 15 seconds.*

Wash your hands before handling your newborn. Of course, you should always wash your hands when preparing food, before feedings, after diapering your baby, and after using the bathroom.

*Source: Centers for Disease Control & Prevention

## The Best Seat in the Car

*To protect your baby, be sure everyone caring for your baby follows this rule...*

Use a rear-facing infant safety seat that is properly installed in the back seat every time your baby rides in a car.

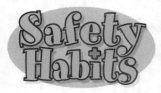
# Homework Before the Baby

• Take a class in infant first aid and CPR, including how to rescue a choking infant.

• Give your baby the gift of a smoke-free environment. Make this a lifelong commitment for your home and family. You'll all live longer.

• Install smoke alarms and begin a monthly habit (every first day of the month) of checking to be sure the batteries are strong and the alarm is working.

• Plan a safe escape route from the room where your baby sleeps. If necessary, buy (and be sure you know how to use) a window escape ladder. Keep a working fire extinguisher on every floor of your home.

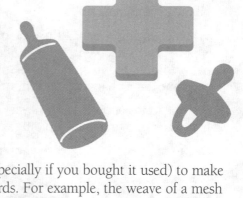

• Reset the hot water heater thermostat so that the water temperature stays below 120° F.

• Check baby's furniture (especially if you bought it used) to make sure it meets safety standards. For example, the weave of a mesh playpen or portable crib should have small (less than 1/4 inch) openings. Your baby's crib should have slats no more than 2-3/8 inches apart, and the mattress should be firm and fit snugly into the crib.

# Your Newborn Baby

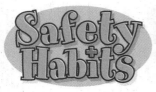

## Home Safe Home

*To protect your baby, be sure everyone caring for your baby knows and follows these rules:*

- Back to sleep! Unless your doctor tells you otherwise, put your baby to sleep on his or her back. This sleeping position reduces your baby's risk of Sudden Infant Death Syndrome (SIDS).

- Be sure the place you put your baby to bed is safe. Your baby should not get too cold or too hot while sleeping. The room temperature should be 65°-68° F. Always keep crib siderails up and latched. Never leave your baby in a playpen or portable crib with the drop-side down. Do not use soft bedding, pillows, comforters, soft toys, toys with loops, or string cords.

- When changing a diaper, dressing baby, or giving your baby a bath, always keep one hand on the baby. Never leave your baby unprotected in a dangerous spot such as in a tub during bathtime, on a changing table, or on a bed or sofa.

- Prevent scalds and burns by never carrying or drinking hot liquids or smoking while holding your baby.

- Don't tempt fate! Never leave your baby alone with a young child or pet.

## Home Safety Shower

Baby gifts that help keep little ones safe are great gifts for babies and parents.

The Consumer Product Safety Commission encourages safety showers by offering information on planning the shower, games and activities to play at the shower, and a 12-point safety checklist for new parents.

A baby safety shower kit may be obtained by calling the Consumer Product Safety Commission at 1-800-638-2772 or by checking out the Web site at *www.cpsc.gov.*

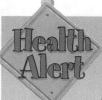
# Fragile, Handle with Care

*To protect your baby, be sure everyone caring for your baby knows and follows this rule…*

**NEVER, NEVER SHAKE A BABY!**
Your baby must never be handled roughly. Sudden, jerking motions such as shaking cause violent back-and-forth movement of the baby's head – and the brain inside the skull.

Bleeding into the brain from torn blood vessels, or swelling of the tissue itself, can result in tragic outcomes – seizures, blindness, deafness, and even death.

Babies must be handled gently to prevent physical and emotional harm. Although every part of your baby's body is fragile, your newborn's relatively large head and weak neck muscles require very special handling. Head support is a "must" while your baby's neck muscles are growing strong enough to hold his or her head without support.

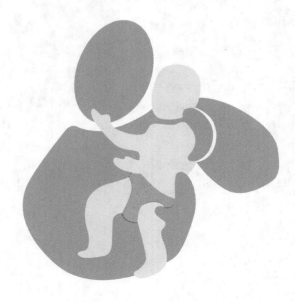

## Physical Growth
### So Big!

Your baby grows more rapidly in the first 6 months than at any other time. Birth weight usually doubles by 4 to 6 months of age. Length usually increases 6 inches or about 1 inch per month in the first 6 months. Head size usually increases by 3 inches.

Your baby's chubby cheeks at 6 months are quite normal. Body fat is added more rapidly than muscle in the 4th and 5th months. Then between 6 and 12 months, your baby will appear to slim down as calories are used to grow strong muscles for walking.

## Eating Well: Birth to 6 Months

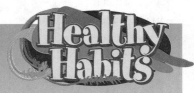

Brain development and physical growth depend on adequate nutrients in adequate amounts – including a diet adequate in fat. **In the first 2 years of life, skim milk and low-fat milk do not provide adequate fat and should not be used in your baby's diet.**

In the first year, breast milk and iron-fortified formulas are good sources of dietary fat. In the second year, whole milk is the appropriate replacement for breast milk or formula.

# Brain Fact

Brain development proceeds at an amazing rate in the first three years of life.

Brain cells branch out to connect with other brain cells – one cell connecting with up to 15,000 others. The connecting branches carry the nerve signals from cell to cell, allowing one brain cell to "talk" with another.

As the connecting branches grow, they are coated with myelin, an insulating covering composed primarily of a type of fat. (See "Healthy Habits, Eating Well" on the previous page.)

# Dental Development
## Baby Teeth

The first teeth (lower front) usually make an appearance at 7 months but are known to arrive as early as 3 months and as late as 12 months.

Family history is a more reliable predictor of the appearance of the first tooth than drooling. The drooling that begins at about 3 months is a sign of salivary glands that are maturing – not teething.

# Books for Your Baby

• Start the habit of reading now.

• Choose brightly illustrated books with stories that rhyme.

• Babies enjoy rhythm and repetition.

• Books that can be grabbed by little hands, chewed on, and read over and over are good investments.

(See "Great Book List" in *Growth and Development Resources*.)

# Birth to 6 Months

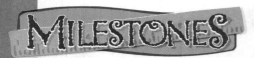 ## Physical Skills

*Usually around 2 months,* babies start their own workout routine to gain head control. When lying on their tummies, babies strengthen the muscles in the back of the neck by head-lifting exercises.

*Usually around 4 months,* babies do "baby push-ups," raising their head and upper body while supporting their weight on their forearms. At this age, babies are using their mouths to explore everything and are taking awkward swipes with their arms at dangling objects. They can shake a rattle placed in their hand and will suck on it if given the chance.

*Usually around 6 months,* babies sit with support and are able to roll from back to tummy. They reach for an object with one hand and are able to transfer it to the other hand. Since they can get both hands to midline, they can now hold their own bottles. When held upright with their feet touching the floor, 6-month-old babies partially support their weight on their legs and may even practice walking movements.

## Play Activities
### Floor Exercises

*How?* Create a wide-open, safe space by placing your baby on a clean blanket on the floor. Get down on the floor and "coach" baby fitness exercises such as gently bicycling baby's legs or placing your baby on his or her tummy for head and chest lifting practice.

*Why?* Practice makes perfect!

# Brain Fact

The areas of the brain associated with smiling mature early, followed by head control, sitting and walking. Identical areas of the brain mature in the same order in all babies, which explains why babies all over the world smile before they have head control and sit before they walk.

# Ask Your Doctor
## Muscle Tone and Strength – 6 Months

Your baby may need developmental evaluation if at age 6 months, he or she:

- seems stiff or floppy
- has difficulty holding up his or her head
- reaches with only one arm or hand
- does not roll over in either direction
- cannot sit well even with support
- does not put hands together

Source: American Academy of Pediatrics
(See First Steps listing in *Growth and Development Resources*.)

# MILESTONES  Language

*Usually around 2 months,* babies recognize and can be comforted by their parents' voices. They begin to "talk" with soft vowel sounds like "aah" and "ooh."

*Usually around 4 months,* babies begin to "babble," repeating vowel sounds and some consonants like "muh-muh-muh" or "bah-bah-bah."

*Usually around 6 months,* babies combine many different sounds to "talk" to you or the "baby in the mirror" in what sounds like adult speech. Babies can tell by the tone of your voice if you are happy, sad, or angry. At this age, they also laugh out loud with a delightful belly laugh.

# Birth to 6 Months

Growth & Development

## Play Activities
### Talking Takes Two – Baby and You

Your baby needs someone who listens, tries to understand and responds. Television and videotapes are not good talking partners.

*How?* If you want to get your baby's attention when you're talking, there's a method that parents all over the world have used for years – baby talk or "parentese." It looks and sounds like this…

- As you speak, look directly at the baby with your eyes open wide, raise your eyebrows and exaggerate your mouth movements.

- Speak in a higher-pitched voice.

- Speak slowly.

- Use a musical voice that gets louder and softer, higher and lower, and starts and stops in a rhythm that sounds almost like singing.

Once you have your baby's attention, watch for signs that your baby wants to participate, such as cooing noises, changing facial expressions, or arm and leg movements. Reward your baby's attempt to enter into the conversation by imitating his or her expressions along with smiles and lots of compliments.

*Why?* Your baby's progress in learning words, how to put words together and how to use words to solve problems depends on you and other caregivers talking to your baby and encouraging your baby to enter into the conversation.

62

# Ask Your Doctor
## Hearing – 6 Months

Your baby may need special testing if at age 6 months, he or she:
- does not respond to loud noises by blinking, crying, becoming quiet, or appearing startled
- does not turn his or her head or eyes toward a voice or noise
- does not respond by smiling (even faintly) at parent's face or voice
- shows no interest in rattles, bells, or noise-making toys
- does not coo or make noises for parents during alert play periods

Source: American Academy of Pediatrics
(See First Steps listing in *Growth and Development Resources*.)

# Emotional Development
## Falling in Love

As you learn to read your baby's moods and needs, comforting your baby becomes easier. You become more sure of yourself and your ability to make your baby happy.

At 3 months, your baby begins to take part in play. Your baby tries in every way possible to tell you he or she is having fun – with waving arms, big smiles, and excited conversations made up of coos, squeals, and giggles.

The time you spend comforting, feeding and playing with your baby helps your baby develop a sense of security. Your baby trusts that you will always be there to meet his or her needs. You become uniquely important to your baby. Your baby becomes securely attached to you.

# Brain Fact

Emotion is the looking glass through which we see the world. Emotion colors every activity, every relationship, and every response. The emotional centers in the brain are so powerful that they can "take charge" of other brain activities like learning.

To learn, your baby must feel secure. Your baby's sense of security depends on trust – trust in you. Without that trust, your baby's learning becomes a prisoner of your baby's emotions. Trust frees up your baby's brain for learning.

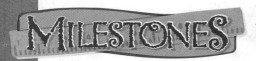

## Learning

The first time your baby smiles, rolls over, says "mama" or "dada," you'll check the date and make a mental note (or record it in a baby book) of the age your baby reached an important milestone. It's easy to observe an activity or to notice a word. It's not as easy to pick up on the progress your baby is making in the areas of learning. "Learning Milestones" will help you appreciate the higher level thinking your baby is doing.

In the first month of life, your baby can imitate simple facial expressions like an open mouth. To do this, your baby must focus on your face and notice your mouth is open. It isn't clear why your baby copies you, but it likely has something to do with your baby trying to make sense of the world.

Toys are important ways to stimulate learning. Mobiles that have simple, bright shapes catch your baby's attention and allow lots of experimenting.

## Brain Fact

At around 3 months, your baby's brain is mature enough to use everyday experiences to make useful discoveries such as learning that kicking the side of the crib makes the animals on the mobile move. Your baby is beginning to understand what scientists call the principle of cause and effect.

## Selecting a Child Care Provider

More than half of all mothers of children younger than 5 years old are employed. If you are a working mother who is taking a maternity leave, you are probably returning to work when you baby is between 6 weeks and 12 weeks old. Although you may find that child care options for infants under the age of 1 year are limited, don't "just make do" when it comes to your baby's happiness or safety.

When evaluating a day care center or a day care home for your baby, make sure there will be no more than three babies for every staff person and that the infants younger than 1 year are cared for separately from toddlers and older children. Choose carefully.

The following guide, "Four Steps to Selecting a Child Care Provider," was developed by the Administration for Children and Families, U.S. Department of Health and Human Services.

For more complete guidelines on health and safety in child care, call the National Resource Center for Health and Safety in Child Care at 1-800-598-KIDS (5437). For the name of the nearest Child Care Resource and Referral Program, call Child Care Aware at 1-800-424-2246. In Indiana, call 1-800-299-1627.

# Four Steps to Selecting a Child Care Provider

## 1. Interview Caregivers

**Call the caregiver and ask these questions:**

- Is there an opening for my child?

- What hours and days are you open? Where are you located?

- How much does care cost? Is financial assistance available?

- How many children are in your care?

- What age groups do you serve?

- Do you provide transportation?

- Do you provide meals (breakfast, lunch, dinner, snacks)?

- Do you have a license, accreditation, or other certification?

- When can I visit?

**Next, visit the child care facility or home; visit more than once and stay as long as you can. Look for these indicators of a healthy environment:**

- Responsive, nurturing, warm interactions between caregiver and children.

- Children who are happily involved in daily activities and comfortable with caregivers.

- A clean, safe and healthy indoor and outdoor environment, especially napping, eating and toilet areas.

- A variety of toys and learning materials that your child will find interesting and that will contribute to growth and development.

- Children getting individual attention.

**Ask the caregiver:**

- How do you handle discipline?
- What do you do if a child is sick?
- What would you do in the case of an emergency?
- What training have you and other staff/substitutes had?
- Are all children and staff required to be immunized?
- May I see a copy of your license or other certification?
- Do you have a substitute or back-up caregiver?
- May I have a list of parents who use or have used your care?
- Where do children nap? Are babies put to sleep on their backs?

## 2. Check References

**Ask other parents who use the caregiver these questions:**

- Is the caregiver reliable on a daily basis?
- How does the caregiver discipline your child?
- Does your child enjoy the child care experience?
- If your child is no longer with the caregiver, why did you leave?
- How does the caregiver respond to you as a parent?
- Is the caregiver respectful of your values and cultures?
- Would you recommend the caregiver without reservation?

**Ask the local child care resource and referral program or licensing office:**

- What regulations should child care providers in my area meet?
- Is there a record of complaints about the child care provider I am considering, and if so, what can I find out about it?

## 3. Make the Decision for Quality Care

**From what you heard and saw, ask yourself these questions:**

- Which child care should I choose so that my child will be happy and safe?
- Which caregiver can meet the special needs of my child?
- Are the caregiver's values compatible with my family's values?
- Is the child care available and affordable according to my family's needs and resources?
- Do I feel good about my decision?

## 4. Stay Involved

**Ask yourself these questions about your child care arrangement:**

- How can I work with my caregiver to resolve issues and concerns that may arise?
- How will I stay informed about my child's developmental accomplishments?
- How can I promote good working conditions for my child care provider?
- How can I network with other parents?
- How can I arrange my schedule so that I can talk to my caregiver every day, visit and observe my child in care at different times of the day, and be involved in my child's activities at the day care?

## Is it a "Good Fit"?

*Watch your baby for signs of a good or bad "fit" with new child care arrangements.*

Signs that suggest things aren't going well for your baby include fewer smiles or clinginess and irritability. Another red flag is a caregiver who shows no delight in your baby – no welcoming smile, no cute stories at the end of the day. If you get the sense your baby is "just another mouth to feed," it's time to find another caregiver.

## Hi Ho, Hi Ho, it's Off to Work You Go

There is no one best time to go back to work, but there are some times that are not so good for your baby.

It's best not to schedule your return to work right after a move or any other break in the daily routine that your baby finds comforting. It's also best to avoid the period around major milestones like walking or toilet training. These are times your baby will want the security of having you close.

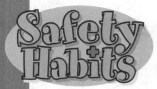

## Child Care for Your Child with Special Needs

In addition to the usual qualities parents look for in child care arrangements, you'll have additional criteria that must be met to be sure you have the right individual and the right facility for your child with special needs. When you interview a child care provider, ask these questions...

- Does the caregiver have experience in caring for a child with similar special needs?

- Is the caregiver trained and certified in rescue skills and first aid?

- Is the caregiver willing to adapt his or her program to meet your child's needs?

- Is the caregiver willing to take responsibility for the necessary medical procedures and medication your child requires?

- Does the facility have enough space for any extra equipment your child requires?

- Are the play materials and toys appropriate for your child?

- Is the site safe for your child? Could your child and necessary medical equipment be transported quickly and easily from the facility in the case of an emergency?

- If increased electrical capacity is necessary for medical equipment, is it available? Is the caregiver willing to make arrangements for emergency power for medical equipment in case of an electrical outage?

*If you need help in finding a quality child care center, contact the Indiana Association for Child Care Resource and Referral at 1-800-299-1627.*

# Home Emergency Planning for Your Child with Special Needs

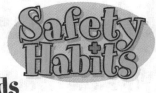

- Notify local emergency services including the electric company of special health care requirements for your child.

- Make arrangements for emergency power for medical equipment in the case of an electrical outage.

- Post an emergency plan for transporting your child and necessary medical equipment from the house in the case of an emergency.

- Practice your home fire escape plan to be forewarned of possible difficulties.

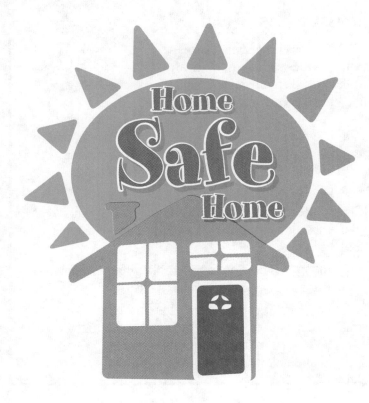

# 6 Months to 1 Year

## Physical Growth
### No Wonder Baby's Hungry!

Your baby's first growth spurt – which began even before birth – lasts until age 2. At 12 months, your child usually weighs around 21 pounds, is around 30 inches long, and measures a head size of about 18 inches.

Boys are slightly heavier and longer than girls at this age.

Body proportions begin to change as "too short" arms and legs begin to "catch up" with the baby's long trunk.

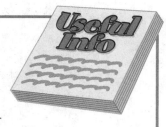

## Your Baby Has Style!

Actually all babies have style – a style of reacting to the world around them. This style is called temperament, and just like brown eyes or curly hair, your baby is born with his or her temperament. Recognizing your baby's unique temperament and adjusting the environment to fit your child is an important responsibility of parenting. Babies are usually described as fitting into one of three temperament categories.

*Easy:* Easy babies eat and sleep on schedule, are usually happy, and accept change easily. Easy babies make parents look and feel good.

*Slow to warm up:* These quiet babies like routines, resist being hurried, and are slow to accept change.

*Intense:* Intense babies are challenged by just about everything. They have trouble sleeping and accepting new foods and tend to be fussy. Intense babies require patience and special handling.

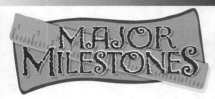
**MAJOR MILESTONES**

# Language

*Around 6 months,* your baby begins to understand a few words. He or she also invents sounds for happiness or other emotions. More and more of your baby's vocalizations sound like speech.

*Around 9 months,* your baby invents words for objects, like "ba" for bottle. Words like "mama" and "dada" said by accident create such excitement that very quickly the sounds transform into real words with meaning.

*Around 12 months,* your baby says his or her first real word. Your baby also responds to "no" and uses simple gestures like waving for "bye-bye" and head shaking for "no."

# A Good Night's Sleep

At about 6 months of age, your baby sleeps all through the night – 11 hours. In addition, your baby takes two naps totaling 3-4 hours during the day. Your baby is resting up for the last month or so of the year when nighttime waking resurfaces.

Between 10 and 18 months of age, your baby is likely to wake in the night and want to see you. Help your baby self-comfort by offering a stuffed toy, a favorite blanket, or a pacifier.

**Useful Info**

# Play Activities!
## Now it's Your Turn

*How?* Use a damp washcloth to wash your baby's hands after mealtime. Offer the washcloth to your child to take a turn washing your hands. You can play "Now it's your turn" with feeding, too. Let your baby take a turn feeding you with a spoon. You'll think of other variations.

*Why?* Babies like to imitate adults, so the game is fun for the baby. It also allows your baby to practice skills that use small muscles and require coordination. You may find that the next time you wash your baby's hands or feed your child, your baby will be more cooperative.

73

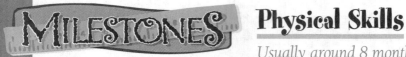 ## Physical Skills

*Usually around 8 months,* your baby sits without support. When your baby lies down, he or she is in constant motion, which makes diaper changes especially dangerous. Some babies begin crawling at this time. Others scoot and some roll to get where they're going.

*Usually around 10 months,* your baby can pull up to standing from a sitting position, can stand holding on to something or someone, can play pat-a-cake, and may be able to pick up tiny objects by using his or her thumb and forefinger.

*Usually around 12 months,* your baby is able to walk while holding on to furniture or using your hands, drink from a cup, pick up a tiny object using the tips of his or her thumb and forefinger, and stand alone for a few seconds.

## Brain Fact

Some babies walk early and some walk late. Parents of early walkers may hope that this is a sign of exceptional intelligence. In fact, there is no relationship between intelligence and the age of walking or other physical skills.

It's good to celebrate every one of your baby's accomplishments, but beware of putting emphasis on the timing. Bright babies may walk early or late. It's just too soon to tell.

# Ask Your Doctor
## Development – 1 Year

Your baby may need developmental evaluation if at 1 year, he or she:

• does not crawl

• drags one side of the body while crawling

• is unable to stand even with support

• does not search for hidden objects

• says no single words

• does not wave goodbye, shake head, or use other gestures

• does not point to pictures or body parts

Source: American Academy of Pediatrics
(See First Steps listing in *Growth and Development Resources.*)

# MILESTONES    Learning

During this developmental period, your child is both an explorer and a scientist.

*Usually around 6 months,* your baby discovers gravity. As your baby's laboratory assistant, your job is to pick up the toys, the food, or the bottle that your baby drops. This is an experiment your baby will repeat over and over again.

*Usually around 9 months,* your baby understands that an object continues to exist even when it is out of sight. If you hide a ball under a blanket, your scientist knows how to make it reappear. Your baby is now able to keep a mental picture of the ball in his or her memory.

*Usually around 12 months,* your baby develops an understanding that objects have names and uses. As a 6-month-old, your baby used pretty much every object as a toy to bang, rattle, or chew. By the end of the first year, your baby understands that a cup is for drinking, a spoon is for feeding, and a rattle is for shaking.

# 6 Months to 1 Year

Growth & Development

## Books for Your Baby

Certain books are extremely popular with children, usually because they do a great job of delivering the right message for the right age in the right way. Many of these books become favorites and become part of the bedtime routine night after night.

There are many reasons a child attaches to a particular book. Some of the most common reasons and popular books are listed below.

- Offers reassurance – *Who's Mouse Are You?* by Robert Kraus
- Easy to identify with – *Sam's Teddy Bear* by Barbro Lindgren
- Humor – *Curious George* by H.A. Rey
- Easy to predict/ Lots of repetition – *Brown Bear, Brown Bear, What do you see?* by Bill Martin, Jr.
- Great pictures – *The Snowy Day* by Ezra Jack Keats
- Pleasing rhythm to the words – *Madeline* by Ludwick Bemelmans
- Happy book – *Blueberries for Sal* by Robert McCloskey
- Uses gimmicks like lift-ups or flaps – *Where's Spot?* by Eric Hill
- Topic of special interest – *Big Wheels* by Anne Rockwell

Favorite books serve a purpose for your child. Once the purpose has been served, your child will be ready to go on to new books. The next time you are re-reading a story for the 100th time, congratulate yourself on helping your child work through the many challenges of childhood.

(See "Great Book List" in *Growth and Development Resources*.)

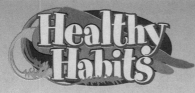

## Toothbrushing

As soon as the first tooth appears, you need to start the habit of cleaning your child's teeth.

Use a clean, moist washcloth to wipe your baby's teeth and gums. Use only water – no toothpaste. A soft, small toothbrush can also be used for baby teeth.

# Emotional Development
## Falling in Love

Two important emotional milestones are reached during the second six months of life.

*Stranger anxiety:* At 6 months, your baby was the life of the party. He or she had smiles for everybody. Strangers complimented you on your socially outgoing child.

About 9 months of age, your baby begins to react differently to strangers. Now your baby is clingy, fussy, and turns away from smiling faces. You may hear comments that you are "spoiling" your child.

Not so! Your 9-month-old saves his or her smile for familiar faces. Your social 6-month-old and your stranger-shy 9-month-old are both right on track in their emotional development.

*Separation anxiety:* Another change occurs at 9 months. Your baby becomes intensely aware of your importance in his or her life. The idea of losing you, even for one minute (especially when your child has no sense of time) is not tolerable. And so your baby cries, clings to you, and generally sounds as if his or her heart is breaking whenever you attempt to separate.

Although you may find this stage difficult, your child's reaction to separation is telling you what a good job you have done. Congratulations! Babies who show no separation anxiety between 10 and 18 months are a cause for concern.

## Brain Fact

Peek-a-boo may be the first "brain game" you play with your baby.

If you play peek-a-boo with your 6-month-old, when you open your hands to show your face, your baby is probably looking somewhere else. To a 6-month-old, you are truly "out of sight and out of mind."

Play peek-a-boo with your 9-month-old and when you open your hands, your child squeals with delight.

This simple age-old game gives you a peek at your baby's understanding that something continues to exist even when it can't be seen – an understanding that indicates the areas for higher level thinking in your baby's brain are becoming active.

## Questions&Answers

Q: Why does my 8-month-old break into tears when I arrive to pick him up from day care?

A: When your baby sees you, he remembers how much he misses you. He can't tell you he missed you, but his tears show the intensity of his feelings.

To help your baby get back in control, spend a few minutes playing with him before preparing to leave for home. When he calms down, he'll be able to remember he enjoys the day care and perhaps he'll show you someone or something that he likes. That will make both of you feel better.

## Say "No" to Baby Walkers

**Health Alert**

*Baby walkers are not safe.*

Each year, there are more than 25,000 injuries from baby walkers. The most common injuries are head injuries, broken arms and legs, and facial injuries.

Walkers allow infants to move too fast and make it easy for them to get into dangerous situations. In addition to placing an infant in danger, walkers may actually delay walking.

## Avoid Unsafe Clothing

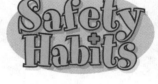

*Flame resistant sleepwear:* Before purchasing, check all sleepwear for a label stating that the clothing item meets the federal government standards for flame resistance. Carefully follow the cleaning instructions to prevent loss of the flame resistant quality. Unless you are sure washing precautions have been followed, don't purchase or accept offers of used sleepwear for your baby.

*Drawstrings or ribbons:* Remove all drawstrings from clothing – hoods, jackets, waistbands. Drawstrings can catch on objects and strangle a child. Cut strings off mittens. Never use a ribbon or piece of string to tie a pacifier to clothing.

*Ribbons and necklaces:* No baby necklaces or pacifiers on ribbon for your baby. Neck ribbons and necklaces can also cause strangulation.

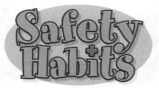

## Teen Babysitters

Be choosy when it comes to hiring a teenage babysitter. Babysitting is a big responsibility. Be sure the person you choose is ready to accept the responsibility for your baby's care, safety, and life.

Ask for recommendations from friends, neighbors, co-workers, or other associates. Look for someone who is experienced. Interview before you hire – in person, if possible. Ask the prospective sitter about:

• experience with children (especially in your child's age group)

• training in first aid and rescue skills (choking)

• training in child care and babysitting skills

• a fair hourly rate

Ask several "what-if" questions, such as,

• "What if my child cries when I leave?"

• "What if someone comes to the door?"

Be sure to check out references. Ask about experience with children of similar age to your child. It is ideal to schedule a one-hour training/observation session (with pay) before the first solo job.

If you are unable to locate a trained teen sitter, you should encourage a prospective sitter to take a babysitter preparation course. Contact your local hospital to determine the availability of babysitter training courses. You can also contact Safe Sitter National Headquarters at 1-800-255-4089 or 317-543-3840 to locate the nearest Safe Sitter training program. You can also visit the Safe Sitter Web site at *www.safesitter.org* for additional information about hiring a babysitter and the Safe Sitter Program.

## Physical Growth
### Lookin' Good!

Your toddler continues to grow steadily. However, after the 2nd birthday, growth slows. By age 2, your toddler weighs four times his or her birth weight, usually measures about 34 inches in length, and has a head size that has grown to almost 90 percent of adult head size.

Between the 2nd and 3rd birthdays, your toddler will usually put on only 3-5 pounds and add only about 3 inches in length.

During the toddler years, the soft, round look of your baby changes. Baby fat begins to disappear from cheeks, arms and legs. Your child develops a neck. Muscles "bulk up" as muscle mass increases twice as fast as bone. Legs are longer and straighter and feet point forward. Your 1-year-old's flat feet develop arches as the fat pad that hid the arch disappears.

# The Toddler Years: 1 & 2

## Brain Fact

During the toddler years, amazing changes are taking place in the brain. The brain is growing in complexity as the number of connections between nerve cells increases to 1,000 trillion, which is twice the number of connections at birth (and twice the number in an adult brain).

In addition, there are three other changes. The supporting cells of the brain multiply. Individual nerves are insulated for more efficient firing, and new blood vessels are formed to supply areas of increased activity with oxygen and nutrients.

## Dental Development
### Baby Your Baby's Teeth

By age 2-1/2, most children have all 20 of their baby or primary teeth. The second molars are the last to appear usually coming in between 20 and 30 months.

Your child's primary teeth are important for chewing, speaking, and your child's smile. Primary teeth are also important for jaw growth. They hold a place for permanent teeth.

Sixty percent of 3-year-olds have one or more cavities. One of the most important things you can do for your child's smile is to take good care of your baby's teeth – regular tooth brushing, a healthy diet, a minimum of sticky, sugary foods and a visit to the dentist.

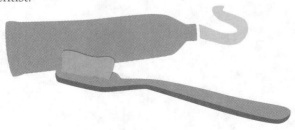

# MILESTONES Physical Skills

*Usually around 18 months,* your child is practicing physical skills every waking hour. You'll be amazed at your child's progress with coordination and balance. Some highlights include walking backwards, walking up stairs holding someone's hand, being able to bend over to pick up a toy, and being able to remove larger pieces of clothing.

*Usually around 24 months,* your child can walk up and down stairs alone and may want to try jumping off the bottom step. Your child can also use a spoon well, kick a large ball, build a tower of six blocks, and unzip a zipper.

*Usually around 36 months,* your child can walk up and down steps alternating feet, can open a door by turning a knob, can bend over easily without falling, and can ride a large wheeled toy like a tricycle. At this age, your child's favorite activity may be running. Get ready!

## Useful Info

## Living with an Intense Toddler

Toddler years are especially challenging for children with intense temperaments. Try these techniques to make life easier for your child (and for you). If your child is:

*Intensely active:* Schedule lots of supervised active play in safe spaces – outside whenever possible.

*Intensely loud:* Ask your child to save loud noises for outdoors and use an "inside voice" when indoors. Encourage singing and reciting nursery rhymes.

(See "Resources: Suggested Books – *The Difficult Child*, by Stanley Turecki, M.D."
in the *Growth and Development* section.)

## Play Activities!
### Daddy Says

*How?* Tell your child to copy your movements. Point to your ear saying, "Daddy says point to your ear." Your child should imitate you. Try pointing to your nose and then your toes, each time saying, "Daddy says point to your nose" or "Daddy says point to your toes." Throw in a few "Daddy says stick out your tongue" or "Daddy says make a funny face" just so you can get your toddler giggling. Don't expect the game to last for more than a few minutes.

*Why?* Toddlers love to imitate, they love activity, and they love having fun, but they have very short attention spans.

## Ask Your Doctor
### Development – 30-36 Months

Your baby may need a developmental evaluation if by his or her 3rd birthday, he or she:

• falls frequently and has difficulty with stairs

• drools or has speech that is difficult to understand

• has difficulty handling small objects

• cannot copy a circle

• doesn't understand simple instructions

• is not interested or has very little interest in other children

• does not have pretend play

• does not put two words together

• is unable to separate from parents without significant protest

Source: American Academy of Pediatrics
(See First Steps listing in *Growth and Development Resources.*)

# MILESTONES

## Learning

During the toddler years, you can almost see your child learning. Your child is able to solve problems by thinking and doing. Your toddler can recognize same and different and begins to have more complicated play. In addition to being able to sort objects by color and shape, your child understands the idea of numbers, especially two.

Toddler years are a time of magical thinking when your child finds it difficult to separate fantasy from reality. Magical thinking can be delightful, for example, a visit from an imaginary friend. It can also be dangerous, for example, a 2-1/2 year old deciding to fly down the steps like Superman.

# Books for Your Toddler

Reading books to your toddler does more than provide entertainment. Sharing books together provides a message that books are important. Reading is a crucial skill for success in school. Help your child get a head start by starting early.

You can tell that your toddler is interested in books if he or she brings you a book to read, tries to hold the book, wants to turn the pages, points at the pictures, asks for the same story over and over, carries a book around the house, or sits and "reads" a book out loud.

(See "Great Book List" in *Growth and Development Resources*.)

# The Toddler Years: 1 & 2

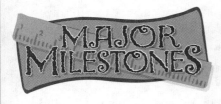

## Language

Mastery of speech and language is perhaps the most variable of developmental milestones. About 1 in every 10 to 15 children has some difficulty with language or speech. Try to be both watchful and reasonable with your expectations. It helps to know that boys usually talk later than girls. Share any concerns you might have with your child's doctor.

Your toddler is better at understanding language than producing it. Children can point to a body part before they can name it.

Some of the most important milestones of the toddler years are imitates animal sounds; refers to self by name; begins to use "I" and "me;" begins to combine words in 2- and 3-word sentences; uses "please" and "thank you;" adds "ed" to verbs to indicate past tense like "I walked" and "s" to nouns to indicate plurals like "dogs;" asks what, where, when and why questions; uses 4 and 5 words in sentences; can be mostly understood by strangers; and understands "on," "in," and "under."

## Brain Fact

A continuing theme in your child's development is the relationship between attachment and achievement. In the first year, your child's eagerness to explore depends on your child's sense of security. In the toddler years, your child's ability to learn depends on feeling secure.

The importance of attachment doesn't go away. In school-age years, children of equal intelligence are most likely to achieve in schoolwork if they have a strong parent-child attachment.

Source: L. Alan Sroufe, Ph.D.

# Emotional Development

Toddlers are incredibly self-centered. You may observe a few of these behaviors: refusing to share, temper tantrums, biting or hitting.

Most toddlers are intense at least part of the time. They can be extremely happy, extremely sad, and extremely angry all within 15 minutes. If your child's temperament is intense, you're likely to see temper tantrums. If your child is quiet, you may see clinginess or whining. It's all part of the same developmental process. Your child is trying to work out how to behave around others. Your help with soothing ruffled feelings and calming angry tantrums is a huge plus for your child's development.

By the time your child reaches 3 years, he or she is able to take turns in games, show affection for playmates, understand "mine" and "his" and "hers," and show more self-control. Your child also begins to show concern for others.

Your child becomes more aware of pleasing or displeasing you during the toddler years. Somewhere around 3, toddlers show emotions such as shame, embarrassment, pride, guilt, and even envy. Self-awareness is a major emotional milestone. Now your child knows that you have expectations and knows whether he or she is living up to them. This is the first step toward the development of conscience.

## Questions & Answers

Q: My first-born took 2-1/2 years to potty train. He wasn't potty trained until 4. With my second-born, I started at age 2-1/2, and he was completely potty trained by age 3. Why?

A: Although there could be lots of reasons why your second-born was easier to potty train than your first-born, here are two possibilities. First, you started the process later with your second-born. Toilet training requires cooperation. Your child has to want to be toilet trained. During the extremely negative period that begins the toddler years, your child doesn't want to cooperate with anything. For that reason, it's best to wait until 2 or 2-1/2 when your child is less negative and more eager to please you. The second reason is your second-born wanted to be grown up like his older sibling.

## Child Rearing Myth

Parents who childproof their homes and who constantly watch their toddlers are being overprotective. Children should learn the rules.

## Child Rearing Fact

Toddlers are too young to be expected to remember and follow the rules. Since toddlers don't have the knowledge or experience to avoid danger or keep their hands off breakables, they require constant watching – especially in a home that hasn't been childproofed.

### Health Alert

## Poison Here! Poison There! Poison, Poison, Everywhere!

*Keep a bottle of syrup of ipecac (non-prescription – costs about $2) on hand and locked in your first-aid kit. Use only on direction of your doctor or the Indiana Poison Center.*

Toddlers are curious. They put everything in their mouths. It's no wonder that 1- to 3-year-olds are at the greatest risk for poisoning. Now that your child can climb, open doors and drawers, and open bottles, everything that could be harmful must be out of sight and out of reach.

You may reach your local poison center by calling 1-800-222-1222 (Universal Poison Center number). See "Poison Safety" in the *Child Safety* section.

# Congratulations!
## You're a Guardian Angel

If there is one time in childhood your child requires a guardian angel, it's the toddler years. Toddlers need constant protection. Be especially watchful when children are hungry, for example, before mealtimes and in the late afternoon. At times of stress or confusion like holidays, family illness, houseguests, or moving day, children are at an increased risk of injury or harm and need extra protection.

# To Grandmother's House We Go

Attention all grandparents. Be sure to enroll in a CPR and first-aid course as soon as you know you'll be grandparents.

Prepare carefully for a visit from your newly walking grandchild – as well as older toddlers and preschoolers. Use the "Room-by-Room Checklist" in the *Child Safety* section to childproof any rooms that will not be kept locked during your grandchild's visit.

More than one-third of all poisonings occur in the homes of children's grandparents. Toddlers will eat anything. Since you can't guard against all the dangers your grandchildren can find, you'll need to take your turn as a guardian angel watching over your little ones.

# Preschool: 3 to 5

## Physical Growth
### Not a Baby Anymore!

Your child's shape changes more than height or weight in the years between the 3rd and 6th birthdays. You can expect your child to add about 4-1/2 pounds and grow about 3 inches each year.

Your preschooler's body "makeover" begins at the top and works down. The bones of the skull and face grow so that your child's face loses some of its roundness, and your child develops a more noticeable forehead, nose and chin. Meanwhile, the upper and lower jaws widen to make room for permanent teeth. The padded shoulder "football player" look of the toddler changes, too. Your child's shoulders narrow, posture improves, and that "toddler tummy" flattens.

Your child's requirement for dietary fat decreases in the preschool years. As your preschooler's body matures, it's time to cut down on high-fat foods like whole milk and cheese. The low-fat diet that is good for you is now good for your child. See "Preschool: 3-5" in the *Nutrition* section.

# Sleep Disturbances

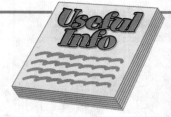

There are several normal sleep behaviors beginning in the preschool years that can be very worrisome to parents

*Sleep Terrors:* Sleep terrors, also called night terrors, may begin as young as age 2. Sleep terrors differ from nightmares. Nightmares are frightening dreams during dream sleep and can be remembered upon awaking. Sleep terrors occur in non-dream sleep and cannot be remembered upon awaking. They usually occur 1 to 4 hours after falling asleep and last between 5 and 30 minutes. They may occur several times in one night or only once in a lifetime. Sleep terrors are far worse for the parents than for the child.

Typically, the child appears to be awake, screams, cries, may thrash, and looks very frightened. Because the child is not fully awake, the child cannot be calmed. When the episode ends, the child returns to full sleep. The good news is children outgrow sleep terrors.

The best way to handle sleep terrors is to stay with your child so that you can protect him or her from any injury caused by thrashing movements. Don't turn on the lights or try to wake your child. Your child will have no memory of the episode. It may help to put your child to bed earlier in case being overtired is contributing to the problem. If the night terrors are very frequent, discuss the problem with your doctor.

*Sleep Talking:* Sleep talking includes talking, laughing, and crying out in sleep. Your child is not aware of what is going on. Even if your child answers your questions, he or she will have no memory of the conversation. Sleep talking is so common it is not considered abnormal.

*Sleep Walking:* Sleep walking may involve only walking or may include a number of other activities, including dressing, raiding the refrigerator, opening doors, and even going up and down stairs. As with night terrors, don't try to wake your child. Gently guide your child back to bed and feel better knowing your child will have no memory of this in the morning.

# Preschool: 3 to 5

*Growth & Development*

## MILESTONES

## Physical Skills

Usually around the age of 3, your child becomes much more coordinated when running or going up and down the stairs. By the end of the preschool years, your child can catch a bounced ball most of the time, kick a ball forward, and stand on one foot or hop. Three-year-olds are so active that sometimes they find it easier to substitute a movement for a word. They may run around the room with their arms spread out to indicate flying instead of talking about flying.

Handedness is well established by age 3. If your child prefers to use his or her left hand, don't try to change it. Lefties do just fine.

Your child's ability to concentrate allows your child to take advantage of the gains in small muscle control in his or her hands. Your child is able to copy a circle and to scribble quite happily. When playing with blocks, your child can build a tower of nine or more cubes.

This is a great age for crafts. Your child loves to practice cutting, painting, and coloring. For future gardeners, it's a great time to work in the garden. For future carpenters, nothing beats the thrill of using a real screwdriver.

Self-help skills are much improved. At this age, children can feed themselves, unbutton their clothes, and handle large zippers and snaps.

# Play Activities!

*How?* Find three pictures that show something happening like a boy riding a bike, falling off, and his mother coming to him. Paste the pictures on to 3 x 5 cards. Ask your child what happened first, next, and last.

*Why?* Practicing placing cards in an order that makes sense will help your child at school.

# Ask Your Doctor
## Development – Almost 5 Years

Your preschooler may need a developmental evaluation if, as the 5th birthday nears, he or she:

- has difficulty throwing a ball overhand
- is unable to jump in place
- is unable to hold a crayon correctly
- is unable to stack four blocks
- won't separate willingly from parents
- is not interested in other children
- is not interested in interactive games
- responds very little to non-family members
- has no imaginative play
- is uncooperative with dressing, sleeping, toilet training
- has difficulty with self-control when angered or upset
- is unable to give his or her first and last name
- does not use plurals or past tense properly
- does not use "me" and "you" correctly
- does not speak in sentences of more than three words
- seems unhappy or sad most of the time

Source: American Academy of Pediatrics

# Preschool: 3 to 5

Growth & Development

## MILESTONES

## Learning/Thinking

Preschoolers continue to use magical thinking to solve problems or explain things. You'll be surprised what you learn when you ask your child a "why?" question. For example, your preschooler may tell you that the sun comes up in the morning because that is when it wakes up.

Sometimes an answer alerts you to a possible problem, such as your child believing that his or her anger could make someone ill. Be firm when you explain that emotions don't cause illness or harm to others.

Preschoolers are not logical thinkers. They believe what their eyes tell them even if it makes no sense. Try this famous experiment with your preschooler to get a better understanding of how your child thinks. Pour water from a tall, thin glass vase into a wide, clear glass bowl. Make sure no water spills. Ask your preschooler which container has more water. Very likely, your child will answer the tall, thin vase (or whichever container appears larger to the child). It's unlikely that your preschooler will say that the amount of water has not changed and it only looks different.

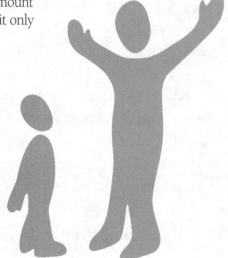

Even if you point out that no water was added or taken away, your preschooler believes what he or she can see and pays no attention to logic. This is called prelogical thinking and is absolutely normal and charming.

94

# Stuttering

One of the common concerns of parents of preschoolers is stuttering. About 1 in 20 children in this age group stutters. Boys are troubled more than girls. Children tend to stutter when they are tired, upset or talking quickly. Stuttering may actually be an unconscious way for your child to hold a space in the conversation until he or she can get the word or sentence out.

Don't call attention to stuttering. Ignore it. Most stuttering goes away on its own, usually within two to three months. If your child stutters, it might help if you talk slower or make a point of sitting down when your child talks to you so that your child will not feel hurried.

Warning signs that your child's stuttering is not likely to be outgrown include your child feeling very self-conscious about stuttering; losing eye contact with the person to whom he or she is speaking while stuttering; frequently repeating words or parts of words; having facial twitches; breathing faster or showing other signs of difficulty in forming words; stuttering for more than six months; or having a family history of a parent or sibling with stuttering problems.

If your child's stuttering is causing behavior or emotional problems or any of the above warning signs are present, discuss the problem with your doctor.

# Preschool: 3 to 5

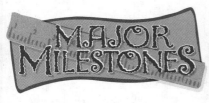

## Language

If you clap for your preschooler's new athletic skills, you should give a standing ovation for the marvelous accomplishments your child is making in language. Consider this:

| Age in years | # Words in vocabulary |
|:---:|:---:|
| 1 | 2-4 |
| 1-1/2 | 10 |
| 3 | 1,000 |
| 5 | 10,000 |

Language is more than vocabulary, however. Words must be combined into sentences. Between the ages of 2 and 5, the number of words in a sentence usually equals the child's age (2-word sentences by age 2, 3-word sentences by age 3 and so on to age 5). Children are also picking up grammar. They practice all these skills by talking and asking questions.

Children learn language at different rates. A number of factors influence language development – first-born children may use language sooner than younger siblings, girls may talk earlier than boys, and children whose parents were late talkers may follow in their parents' footsteps. Active children may be too busy to slow down for a conversation.

The best way to encourage language is by talking and listening to your child – in the car, at the store, at the park, while you're eating, and when you're reading a bedtime story to your child. Talk – listen – talk – listen, etc.

# Brain Fact

A baby's brain comes ready-made with a "blueprint" for learning language. Babies learn words by listening and imitating. But, they learn grammar by paying attention to language and by creating rules that seem to fit.

Since all preschoolers make the same kind of mistakes with grammar, it makes sense that human brains share the same language blueprint. For example, children recognize that by adding an "s" to a word, it becomes plural. So naturally they come up with a word like "mouses." Or by adding "ed" to a word, the word becomes past tense. Using this rule, preschoolers create words like "bringed" and "catched."

Another common problem children have is using pronouns correctly. To avoid the problem of deciding when to use "I" or "me," children frequently substitute their own name for the pronoun. Parents contribute to this problem by avoiding pronouns in sentences such as "Mommy has to take care of baby now."

## School Readiness

Your child is ready for school if he or she knows first and last name; knows home address and phone number; can follow simple instructions; plays well with other children and knows how to take turns; can separate from parents for the time period of a school day; dresses without help; and can use the bathroom without help.

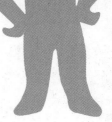

# Questions & Answers

**Q:** My 3-year-old daughter repeatedly steals her new baby sister's blanket. Even worse, she lies and says the baby gave her the blanket. Do I have a juvenile delinquent in the making?

**A:** Preschoolers, especially 3-year-olds, are too young to have an adequate understanding of either truth or ownership to justify being labeled as a liar or a thief. Preschoolers have great difficulty with self-control, and they may take something that they want on impulse. They learn the error of their ways from your negative reaction.

Your child's explanation for taking the blanket is an explanation that comes from her magical thinking and her imagination. In the situation of a new baby, it's likely your little one likes the baby's blanket and hasn't yet learned that wanting it doesn't make it hers. This behavior is typical for a 3-year-old.

The next time you give the blanket back to the baby, remind your preschooler that she has her blanket and the baby has a blanket. The baby can't have her blanket and she can't have the baby's blanket. You'll be helping your child learn an important concept about ownership.

It's best not to pay too much attention to your child's cover-up story. By the time she is 5, she'll understand the difference between something that is true and something that she wants to be true.

# Emotional Development

Preschoolers face several challenges in the area of emotional development.

Preschool years are a time of role-playing. Girls become interested in makeup, nail polish and dress-up clothes. They may become interested in fashion dolls. Boys tend to be interested in cars, trucks and action figures with military or space war themes. Girls tend to play "mommy," and boys tend to play "dad." Role-play is practice for the future.

Your child may have difficulty distinguishing between fantasy and reality. Imaginary friends may come to stay for a while. They usually disappear on their own, replaced by "flesh and blood" playmates. Unfortunately, imaginary monsters are also common at this age and are particularly bothersome at bedtime. Nightlights and reassurance go a long way toward helping your child overcome those fears.

As your child nears age 5, playmates become increasingly important. Your child begins to notice the way that other families do things, which can lead to requests for more privileges and trendy clothing or toys. Your child may experiment with swearing. All of these behaviors are signs that your child is trying to become independent. Your reaction to unacceptable behaviors should separate the behavior from the child. For example, the behavior is "bad," not the child.

Preschoolers are quite aware of sexuality and may ask questions like "Where do babies come from?" This is also a time when children discover and sometimes "play" with their own bodies.

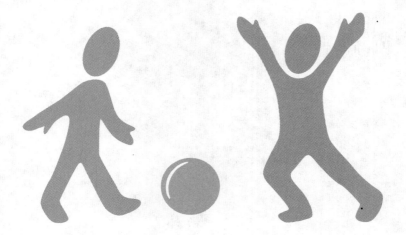

# Preschool: 3 to 5 Safety

*Growth & Development*

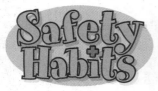

## Preparing Your Child to Go Out into the World

Safety in the preschool years provides another parenting challenge. Early on, you mastered the fine art of babyproofing. During the toddler years, you earned your halo as a guardian angel. Now it's time to take on the responsibility of teaching your child the responsibility of staying safe. In the toddler years, your teaching consisted of warnings like "hot," "don't touch," and "no." In the preschool years, it's time to teach and enforce safety rules.

## The Fabulous Five for Teaching Safety Rules

1. *Set the rules.*

2. *Enforce the rules.*

3. *Be consistent.*

4. *Be reasonable.*

5. *Be firm.*

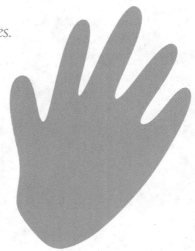

# The Fabulous Five for Helping Preschoolers Learn

1. *Keep it simple.* Think about the safety rules you remember from your childhood. "Look both ways before you cross the street." "Stop, drop, and roll." "Buckle up." It helps to make rules as simple as possible and, when possible, to repeat them using the same words.

2. *Repetition is the glue of learning.* Repeat. Repeat. Repeat.

3. *Learning can be as easy as playing a game.* Teach preschoolers safety rules by playing "what-if" games. First, teach the rule in simple words, and then ask your child a "what-if" question. For example, a fire safety rule for matches and lighters is: "Don't touch. Tell an adult." The "what-if" game question might be: "What if you found a lighter at Uncle Jim's? What would you do?" The preschooler should respond, "Don't touch. Tell an adult." Preschoolers like "what-if" games. They like to get the answer right, and they like to hear you praise them for their correct answers.

4. *Success makes success.* In addition to praising your child for correct answers in the "what-if" game, praise your child whenever you see him or her using good safety habits. If your preschooler holds onto the handrail when going down the stairs, praise him or her for good safety habits on the stairs. Catch your child doing something right as often as possible so that you'll have plenty of opportunities for praise.

5. *Be a good role model.* Your preschooler wants to be just like you when he or she grows up. Everything you do is being watched, so do things right! Make the rule. Teach the rule. Follow the rule – every time.

# School-Age: 6 to 11

## Physical Growth
### Mirror, Mirror, on the Wall...

Before starting school, your child probably had little interest in stepping on the scale or standing by a tape measure. That changes when kids begin to compare themselves with school friends. It may help both of you to know that between the ages of 6 and 11, your child will likely gain an average of 6-7 pounds each year, grow a little more than 2 inches each year, and increase head size by about 1 inch.

The new inches or pounds are added in "mini" growth spurts, usually lasting several months and occurring several times a year.

It's normal at this age for adenoids and tonsils to be large – in fact, tonsils may actually meet in the midline.

The truly attention-getting change in your child will probably be associated with the first signs of puberty. For girls, breast development may start as early as 8 years, although 10 is the average. For boys, enlargement of the testicles and thinning and reddening of the scrotum, (the pouch of skin that holds the testicles) marks the beginning of puberty. Male puberty may begin as early as 9, although 11 is the average.

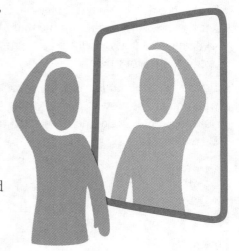

During these years, children of the same age are frequently at different points in their growth and sexual development.

# Questions & Answers

**Q:** What can I give my 10-year-old son to get him eating so he'll grow? He is healthy and active. A few months ago, he grew like a weed, but he was eating then.

**A:** Your son's height depends more on the genes he inherited than the food he eats. When your child is growing rapidly, you can expect him to have a big appetite. When his growth slows, his appetite decreases because he doesn't need the calories. It's not unusual for growth spurts and large appetites to alternate with slow growth and small appetites. Encouraging your son to eat more than he is hungry for will not make him grow, but it may cause him to have a weight problem.

## Useful Info

## Sleep Requirements

With each passing birthday, your child will require a little less sleep. Some kindergarten children need 12 hours of sleep, but most require 10. By age 11, most children can get by with eight hours of sleep. The test is daytime sleepiness.

Bedtime routines, such as a bedtime story or reading in bed for a half-hour before "lights out" can help your child relax. Although bedtime can be an ideal time for a heart-to-heart chat, avoid stressful topics to prevent sleep disturbances.

# School-Age: 6 to 11

## MILESTONES  Learning/Thinking

School-age children have replaced magical thinking and prelogical thinking with concrete logical thinking. If you repeat the experiment on page 94 with a group of children at this age, they are able to answer logically rather than being confused by appearances.

A number of other mental processes are required for success in school. Children need to be able to sequence or put things in order and have an understanding of time. School-age children need to be able to pay attention for fairly long periods of time (45 minutes by age 9) and filter out all unimportant distractions. They also need to develop tricks for memorizing and recalling information on demand.

## Useful Info  Sports, Hobbies, & Exercises

To help your child find an activity that fits his or her interests and talents, provide your child with a wide variety of experiences. Encourage your child to participate in introductory programs offered by your local parks department, YMCA, or other youth organizations. Ask friends or relatives if your child can tag along on a fishing trip, golf outing, or to an antique show if you believe it would be of interest. Once your child settles on a sport or hobby, encourage your child to set personal goals for success and help your child develop the self-discipline to improve.

# Brain Fact

The first 12 years of life are prime time for learning. Experiences actually change the structure of the brain.

During early childhood, the developing brain is busy forming multiple connections between nerve cells. These connections function like the "wiring" of a computer. Each new experience results in a new connection.

By age 3, the child's brain has twice as many connections as an adult's. Connections that are used repeatedly become very strong. Connections that are used infrequently are eliminated. This "use it or lose it" principle is Mother Nature's way of helping each child adapt to his or her own environment.

When connections are eliminated, the ability to perform a particular function is easily lost. For example, in the first months of life, an infant is able to distinguish several hundred spoken sounds, many more than in any single language. As the infant adjusts to his or her native language, the connections for sounds not used in that language are eliminated. The infant can no longer recognize such sounds.

Japanese children who learn English in the first years of life can recognize the difference between "la" and "ra" and are able to pronounce words such as "rice" without difficulty. Whereas a Japanese adult learning English is unable to distinguish "la" and "ra" regardless of exaggerating sounds or slowing speech. The connections to distinguish between "la" and "ra" are gone.

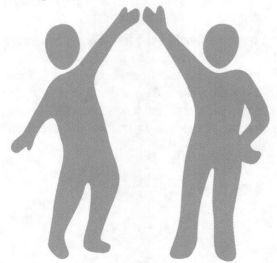

# Top 12 Facts
## You Should Know about Middle Childhood

1. The first mission of middle childhood is to sustain self-esteem – to feel good about oneself most of the time. School years are like an obstacle course for self-esteem. In a single day, a student can experience success, failure, popularity, loneliness, stress, and humiliation. Friends, family and respected adults can help in tough times – so can a history of success in academics or achievement in athletics. However, the most important factor influencing a child's ability to "bounce back" after a bad experience is the presence of at least one parent or adult in the child's life with whom the child has a loving, trusting relationship.

2. The second mission of middle childhood is to be liked and accepted by peers. The desire to be an "insider" and socially accepted is very strong – strong enough to cause children in middle childhood to dress, talk and act as if they had no will of their own.

3. The third mission of middle childhood is to find a way to be like everyone else and, yet, to be different. Most children are able to handle this conflict by modifying their own preferences to "fit in" with the group without completely giving up on all individuality. This mission is often in conflict with mission number 2.

4. The fourth mission of middle childhood is to find acceptable role models for the future. Role models may be selected from television, the music industry, relatives, or even historical or fictional figures. Role models usually come and go as the child ages. Each role model offers the chance to "try on" an identity and a set of behaviors. This mission is helpful for self-discovery and for determining lifetime goals.

5. The fifth mission of middle childhood is to begin the process of questioning the beliefs and values of the family. As children spend increasing time away from home – at school, friends' homes, social events – they realize that there are many differences between values and beliefs learned within their family circle and the values and beliefs of other families. This realization leads to rethinking previously accepted "truths" and starts the child on the path of developing a personal philosophy.

6. The sixth mission of middle childhood is to earn a position of respect within the family. Children want to impress their parents and to gain the respect of the family. This can lead to intense sibling rivalry. A comparison with siblings encourages competition, which can be harmful to both children. Parents must be aware of the importance of acknowledging each child with praise for real achievement. False praise can also be harmful. In addition to the child wanting the respect of parents and family, the child also wants to be proud of his or her family. Family pride is essential to self-worth.

7. The seventh mission of middle childhood is to explore independence and test limits. In the early school-age years, children put up little resistance to parental authority. As the child becomes older, the child becomes more interested in independence and unwilling to accept limits such as curfews or clothing restrictions. The minor conflicts with parents during these years allow the child to rehearse for the role of adolescent and to test his or her ability to handle independence.

8. The eighth mission of middle childhood is to acquire knowledge and master new skills. For a child who learns easily, this mission is a source of reward and pride. For the child who has learning difficulties, this mission offers challenges to self-esteem. Because children of this age have few defenses against failure, a child having learning difficulties often gives up rather than risk being humiliated.

9. The ninth mission of middle childhood is to accept one's own physical appearance, body build, and athletic abilities. If there are two children in this age group in one room, they will be comparing themselves to each other, sure of their own personal defects and bodily abnormalities. The concern school-age children have about their bodies results in extreme modesty, refused invitations to social events like swimming parties, and a great deal of worrying about required showers after physical education classes.

10. The 10th mission of middle childhood is to deal with multiple fears. One of the most common fears in school-age children is fear of the future – worrying about what comes next, possible failures, or humiliation. Another common fear is fear of loss – of family, friends, or even favorite possessions.

11. The 11th mission of middle childhood is to take control of drives and desires. School-age children have an enormous number of "burning desires." To deal with their wants and passions, school-age children must be able to compromise, settle for less than what they had asked for, and accept substitutes or replacements.

12. The 12th mission of middle childhood is to develop a realistic sense of self. By age 12, middle childhood youngsters are usually able to list the things they're good or bad at and their strengths and weaknesses. Children who are able to develop a realistic self-image are most likely to deal well with the challenges of adolescence.

Adapted from Levine, M. *Developmental-Behavioral Pediatrics*. 3rd edition

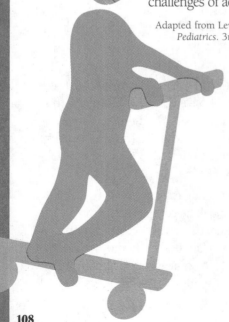

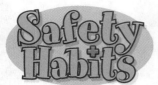

# Home Alone

Sooner or later all parents begin to wonder, "Is it safe to leave my child home alone?" There is no one age when every child is mature enough to handle the responsibilities of staying safe and taking care of oneself. Some children are ready as early as 11, others as late as 15. Use these questions to help think through the various considerations. Begin with the question, "Does my child want to stay home alone?"

## Ability and skills

- Can my child lock and unlock the door?
- Can my child speak clearly on the telephone when providing information or answering questions?
- Can my child prepare a snack?
- Does my child follow directions and remember them for future use?
- Can my child read and write notes?
- Does my child stay interested in productive activities without adult supervision?
- Is my child good at problem solving?
- Does my child handle unexpected situations well?
- Does my child know when to ask for help?

## Safety considerations

- Can my child reach me in an emergency?
- Does my child know when it's important to call local emergency numbers and how?
- Does my employer allow me to make and receive personal calls to check on my child's safety?
- Is there a back-up person if I can't be reached?
- Does my child know basic first aid and rescue skills?
- Do we live in a neighborhood where my child is safe and feels comfortable?
- Does my child know fire escape plans, route, and designated meeting place outdoors?
- Can my child operate appliances such as the stove, microwave, and refrigerator in a safe manner?

# School-Age: 6 to 11 Safety

*Emotional maturity*

- Is my child confident? Fearful? Easily stressed? Easily influenced by peers?
- Does my child use good judgment?
- Does my child have the self-discipline to resist temptation and follow rules without supervision?

*If your child is interested in staying home alone and if he or she appears to have the maturity, then it's time for a training session or two. Make sure your child can do the following things...*

- Locate the emergency numbers. Practice emergency phone calls.
- Execute the home fire escape plan (see "Fire Safety" in *Child Safety* section).
- Contact you or your back-up immediately.
- Perform CPR and first aid (see "Be Ready to Rescue" in Choking Safety of the *Child Safety* section).
- Locate the first-aid kit.
- Answer the phone safely without giving out personal information.
- Handle a delivery or stranger who comes to the door without allowing entry into the home.
- Practice kitchen safety, including use of microwave and practices safe food preparation.
- Handle household emergencies like a power outage or toilet overflowing.
- Lock and unlock the doors and can handle the alarm system.
- Handle other responsibilities that are important in your home, such as pets.

*It is important to establish rules for our child. You can add to the following:*

- Check in with parent immediately after getting home.
- Do not invite friends to visit.
- Do not leave home without permission.
- Begin homework within a half-hour after arrival – after the check-in call and a snack.
- Follow all safety rules.
- Limit television to one hour (or whatever guideline you feel is reasonable).
- Limit computer play time (including video games) to one hour (or whatever guideline you feel is reasonable).
- Follow other rules that are appropriate to your home.

## A word to the wise

There are a number of other precautions to consider. V-chips that block programs inappropriate for children are available in newer television models. Check your television's instruction manual. If your television does not have a V-chip, check with your local electronics or appliance store for information about possible installation of the device.

If you have a computer, you might want to consider blocking access to specific Web sites, such as those that may be too mature for young eyes or chat rooms and bulletin boards where dangerous people may lurk. Check your computer program manual and with your Internet service provider for assistance.

Telephones can also be programmed to block calls with specific telephone number prefixes that are associated with inappropriate call-in lines. Check with your telephone service provider for more information about blocking such calls.

Be sure your child knows to keep the house key out of sight and safe and where to locate a spare key in an emergency.

# A Letter to Parents...

*As your child approaches the teen years, especially if it's your first-born, you find yourself paying attention to the tattoos, body piercing, and clothes of the teenagers you see on the street or in the mall. The realization that your child will soon be "one of them" makes the future seem a little scary.*

*To bolster your confidence for the days ahead, you focus on the strength of your family ties. You wonder if your family will be protected from the problems others have had with their teens by all the hours you invested in providing transportation, helping with homework, attending recitals, cheering at ball games, the fun of family vacations and holiday celebrations. You find yourself thinking back to the "terrible twos" and wondering if the teen years are just a replay. If the toddler years were easy, you hope you'll be lucky with adolescence, too. Although you know it's just a fairy tale, you find yourself wishing for the magic spell in Sleeping Beauty so that your child can sleep peacefully through the teen years and wake up an adult.*

*You have expectations for what's about to happen to you, your child, and your family – as does your child. Your expectations are based on your observations of other families, your understanding of this developmental stage, and your own experience as a teenager. There will be times you will be tempted to share your "I had it much worse than you" and "I know exactly what you're going through" stories with your teen. Proceed with caution. Your stories are your stories. To your teenager, your experiences don't seem relevant and, even worse, they imply that you don't give your teen credit for being a unique individual with his or her problems or concerns.*

*The information on the next few pages has been collected to help you during the years of parenting your teenager. There are also helpful resources at the end of this section. Before moving ahead, however, we suggest you revisit the past. Even though it's unlikely to help your child relate better to you, it may help you relate better to your child. Recalling the intense emotions and pressures you had as a teenager might make it easier to live with, love, support, and champion your child through this dramatic and wonderful passage to adulthood.*

*Have a safe journey.*

# Parents: Test Your Memory!

Instructions: Take this test each year on your child's 11th to 17th birthdays. Think back to the year you were your child's age. Picture yourself in front of a mirror before an "important" event. Let the person in the mirror do the talking. (Honest answers are correct.)

|  | Yes | No | I can't decide |
|---|---|---|---|
| 1. I like the way I look. | ☐ | ☐ | ☐ |
| 2. I feel confused about what's going on with my body. | ☐ | ☐ | ☐ |
| 3. I hate when my family discusses my private business. | ☐ | ☐ | ☐ |
| 4. I don't have enough privacy. | ☐ | ☐ | ☐ |
| 5. I hate being nagged about eating, sleeping, what I wear, cleaning up after myself, my friends. | ☐ | ☐ | ☐ |
| 6. Sometimes I feel lonely, even when I'm with my friends. | ☐ | ☐ | ☐ |
| 7. I hate walking by a group of kids. I know they talk about me. | ☐ | ☐ | ☐ |
| 8. Sometimes I feel so stressed, I think of running away. | ☐ | ☐ | ☐ |
| 9. I know some kids who use drugs, and they seem like they're OK. | ☐ | ☐ | ☐ |
| 10. There's no way to avoid parties where kids are drinking. | ☐ | ☐ | ☐ |
| 11. I've tried smoking, and I can take it or leave it. | ☐ | ☐ | ☐ |
| 12. My friends seem to drive fine when they're drunk. | ☐ | ☐ | ☐ |
| 13. If no one else in the car is using a seatbelt, I don't either. | ☐ | ☐ | ☐ |
| 14. I've heard of a lot of ways that you can have sex without using condoms or contraceptives and not get pregnant. | ☐ | ☐ | ☐ |
| 15. I can't know what to do with my life. I don't even know what's out there. Graduating seems like falling off a cliff. | ☐ | ☐ | ☐ |
| 16. I'm a lot smarter than my test scores and grades show. | ☐ | ☐ | ☐ |
| 17. These are the years to play. I have to work the rest of my life. | ☐ | ☐ | ☐ |
| 18. My parents don't really understand what it's like to be my age. | ☐ | ☐ | ☐ |
| 19. Someone in my family is always mad or complaining about something. I wish they would "get it together." | ☐ | ☐ | ☐ |
| 20. When I'm too old for fun, I'll eat right, exercise, and get sleep. | ☐ | ☐ | ☐ |

# Adolescents: 12 to 21

## Top 10 Facts
### You Should Know about Adolescence

1. Adolescence is the developmental stage between childhood and adulthood. It is more than physical growth and sexual maturation (puberty or biological development). Adolescence includes dramatic and important changes in thought processes of the brain (intellectual or cognitive development) and changes in the way the teen thinks of himself/herself and relates to others (psychosocial or social/emotional development).

2. The age that puberty begins and ends – and how fast the process goes – can be very different for different individuals and still be normal. Puberty in one girl can start as early as age 8 and proceed to menstrual periods by the time she is 10; while another girl starts breast development at age 11 and does not start menstruating until she is 14.

3. It is normal for development to proceed steadily for a while and then stop for a few months. This can be especially troubling when a short male grows quickly for a few months and then stops just when his hopes are up.

4. The three areas of development (physical/sexual, intellectual, and social/emotional) do not necessarily progress at the same rate. This can be troubling for a girl whose sexual development occurs early, making her appear "grown up," but her social/emotional development is still that of a child; or for a teenage boy who has his growth spurt early, making everyone expect him to act his "height age" – not his chronological age.

5. There are three stages of adolescence. Early adolescence – the middle-school years: 11, 12, 13, 14. Middle adolescence – the high-school years: 15, 16, 17. Late adolescence – the age of maturity: 18, 19, 20, 21. Each stage is associated with specific characteristics.

6. There are four developmental goals for adolescence: to become independent of family; to form close, personal relationships; to become comfortable with body and self-image; and to develop an individual identity, realistic life goals, the life skills to "get on" in the world and settle on personal, moral, religious, and sexual values. These four goals are accomplished stepwise as the child goes through the three stages of adolescence – early, middle, and late.

7. Early adolescence (11, 12, 13, 14) is the time of the dramatic physical changes of puberty. Early work on developmental goals begins in this stage. *Independence:* not as willing to do things with family; moody. *Friends:* form close friendships with teens of the same sex, usually one best friend. *Body/self-image:* worried about being normal, attractive; preoccupied with concerns about sexual maturation, including wet dreams and masturbation. *Individual identity:* feel watched; daydream; plan for the future although not necessarily realistic plans; begin to test limits; think about sex, which may lead to masturbation or wet dreams; lack impulse control; exaggerate personal problems out of proportion.

8. Middle adolescence (15, 16, 17) is the time of intense emotions and intense relationships with peers. *Independence:* argue with parents more than any other stage; turn to friends – not parents – for support. *Friends:* want to fit in with chosen peer group, including clothing, values, music; dating and sexual experimentation begin; may get involved in clubs, gangs, and other groups. *Body/self-image:* more comfortable with physical changes; physical attractiveness is important. *Individual identity:* consider the feelings of others; capable of more difficult thought processes; more realistic plans for the future; magical thinking about being able to take risks and not be harmed.

9. Late adolescence (18, 19, 20, 21) is the last step to adulthood. It can be a depressing time if the goals for early and middle adolescence were not successfully reached. *Independence:* become closer to family again; more likely to accept advice. *Friends:* less dependent on group activities; more time spent in meaningful relationship with one partner. *Body/self-image:* OK with body. *Individual identity:* develop practical, realistic career goals; able to compromise; settle on personal, moral, religious, and sexual values.

10. The 21-year-old who is socially and emotionally independent of parents while still close to them, who is comfortable with himself/herself as an adult, and who is capable of meaningful relationships has successfully completed the passage from childhood to adulthood.

**115**

# Adolescents: 12 to 21

## Physical Growth

Growth during adolescence is linked to the hormonal changes of puberty. Girls usually enter puberty earlier than boys.

*Girls*

The age that your daughter enters puberty depends on several factors including her general health, her nutritional status, and family history.

You can predict the order of the changes associated with puberty, but you can't predict the timing. Girls usually develop breast buds before pubic and axillary hair. About two years later, menstrual periods begin. A growth spurt begins before breast budding and ends before periods begin.

*Boys*

You can predict the order of the changes associated with puberty, but you can't predict the timing. Boys usually begin puberty with enlargement of the testicles and scrotum. Pubic hair begins to grow. At the same time, boys may begin to ejaculate. The penis becomes longer and thicker. At the same time, hair grows on the face and underarms and the voice deepens. A growth spurt begins at the same time pubic hair appears and usually lasts 24 to 36 months.

### Useful Info

### Growing Like a Weed

Teens are more likely to shoot up in height in the spring and summer. Hands and feet grow first, followed by arms and legs, and finally chest and trunk.

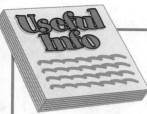
**Useful Info**

# See How They Grow

The inches and pounds added during adolescence count in a big way.

Inches added to height = 25 percent of final adult height

Pounds added to weight = 50 percent of final ideal weight

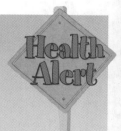
**Health Alert**

# When Puberty Comes too Early

Call your doctor for an appointment for the following:

*Girls*
Before age 7-8: Breast development or pubic hair

Before age 10: Menstrual periods

*Boys*
Before age 9: Enlargement of the testicles and scrotum or pubic hair

# When Puberty Comes too Late

Call your doctor for an appointment for the following:

*Girls*
At age 13: No signs of breast enlargement

At age 16: No menstrual periods

*Boys*
At age 14: No testicular enlargement

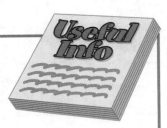

## What You and Your Daughter Should Know about Breast Cancer

- Routine self-examination of the breast should be taught at puberty.

- Cancer of the breast is unusual before age 25. However, over an entire lifetime, 1 in 8 women will have breast cancer.

- A history of a sister or mother with breast cancer increases the risk of cancer.

- Breast cancer is most often discovered during self-examination.

- When discovered by a routine self-exam, breast cancer usually has a better outcome.

- Routine self-exams make early discovery of a change from normal shape or feel of the breast more likely.

- Once a month (at the end of her menstrual period), your daughter should check each breast for a lump that is firm and nonmovable, a dimple on the skin, a change from the normal shape or feel, or discharge from the nipple. The most common place for breast cancer is under the nipple and in the upper fourth of the breast above the nipple and on the side toward the armpit.

- Ask the doctor to show your daughter how to do a self-exam.

- Be sure your daughter knows the signs that require prompt evaluation – a lump that is firm and nonmovable, a dimple on the skin, a change from the normal shape or feel, or discharge from the nipple.

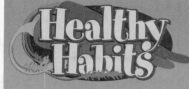

# How to Perform a Breast Self-Exam

The exam is easiest to perform during a shower or bath when the skin is soapy, making a lump easier to feel as your fingers slide over the slippery skin. It is normal to feel the glandular portion of the breast in the shape of a comma with the "tail" of the comma leading up from the center of the breast to the underarm area.

1. Using your flattened fingers, feel for lumps or tenderness beginning with the area under the nipple and moving outward to cover the entire breast in a circular pattern. (Do not use the tips of your fingers since they are too sensitive and can mistake the uneven texture of normal breast tissue for lumps.) Check for areas where the skin of the breast feels "stuck" to the tissue under it. (You may see a dimple or a pucker over this area when you look in the mirror.)

2. Gently squeeze each nipple to check for discharge.

3. Call your doctor for an appointment if you find a firm, nonmovable lump, a dimple on the skin, a change from the normal shape or feel, or discharge from the nipple. Do not check and recheck the abnormal finding. Leave it alone and see a doctor.

4. Do not put off your call to the doctor hoping the problem will go away on its own.

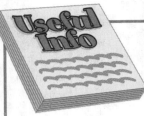

# What You and Your Son Should Know about Cancer of the Testis

- Routine self-examination of each testis should begin at age 13 or 14.
- Cancer of the testis is the most common solid tumor of young men.
- Cancer of the testis is most often discovered during self-examination.
- When discovered early, cancer of the testis is highly curable.
- A history of only one testis or an undescended testis increases the risk of cancer. Both the surgically "brought down" testis and the normally descended testis are at increased risk for cancer.
- Once a month, your son should check each testis for a lump, increase in size, or unusual tenderness.
- Ask the doctor to show your son how to do a self-exam.
- Be sure your son knows the signs that require prompt evaluation – a lump, increase in size, or unusual tenderness.

## Sudden Groin Pain

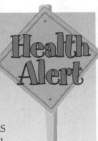

*Seek care immediately for sudden "knife-like" groin pain (frequently so severe there is nausea and vomiting) in males age 12 and older.*

The most common cause of sudden groin pain in this age group is testicular torsion or twisting of the blood supply to the testis. Emergency surgery within four to six hours is required to prevent permanent damage to the testis.

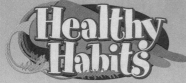

## How to Perform a Testicular Self-Exam

The exam is easiest to perform after a shower when the skin of the scrotum is relaxed. It is normal to feel a soft bumpy area on the top and behind the testis – this is the epididymis. The firm, rope-like structure on the back and above the testis is the vas deferens.

1. Holding the testis between your thumb and fingers, roll the testis between your fingers feeling for lumps or unusual tenderness. Check to be sure there is no difference in size between the two testes.

2. Call your doctor for an appointment if there is an abnormal or questionably abnormal finding. Do not check and recheck the abnormal finding. Leave it alone and see a doctor.

3. Do not put off your call to the doctor hoping the problem will go away on its own.

## Questions&Answers

**Q:** My 14-year-old son has what feels like a rubbery, movable lump under his right nipple. Could he have breast cancer?

**A:** In early puberty, it is not uncommon for boys to have a lump or nodule beneath one or both nipples. A nodule may or may not be painful. These nodules usually disappear within 12 to 18 months as male hormone levels increase. There is no reason to be concerned about breast cancer.

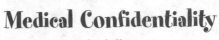

## Medical Confidentiality

*"But I pay the bill"*

During adolescence, it is appropriate for your teen to take an active role in his or her personal health and medical care. Until now, your child's health was your responsibility. In adolescence, most of that responsibility shifts to your teen.

By accepting an adult responsibility, your teen earns the right to doctor-patient confidentiality. Confidentiality is important for open, honest communication. Your teen must trust that private conversations will remain private – off limits even to you!

There are situations in which your doctor learns information that cannot be kept in confidence. For instance, if your doctor learns that a life is in danger, such as a possible suicide attempt, your doctor will inform you so that together, you can take the steps necessary to prevent a tragedy.

Your teen's physician knows you are extremely concerned about your child's well-being. If you feel the need to discuss your concerns or ask for parenting advice, consider requesting an appointment for a parenting consultation.

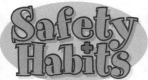

## In Case of an Auto Accident

Be sure your teen knows what to do if involved in a motor vehicle accident. Stress the importance of remaining at the scene. Write out simple directions on a 3 x 5 card (including insurance information) and place it in the glove compartment of the car, along with auto registration.

# It's the Law!

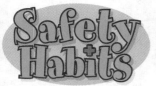

Under usual circumstances, the parent/legal guardian must provide consent for medical care of a minor considered by law to be a person under age 18. However, the State of Indiana authorizes minors to consent for their own medical services under certain conditions. These include: emergency care for a life-threatening condition; examination and treatment for sexually transmitted diseases, including HIV and AIDS; and evaluation and treatment for alcoholism or alcohol or drug abuse at a facility approved by the Division of Addictive Services.

Although the State of Indiana does not directly address the legal rights of minors regarding medical consent for contraceptive services, that right is indirectly assumed under federal case law.

## Safety Habits

## Just in Case...

Chances are the police will stop your teen for a motor vehicle violation sometime in the teen years. Because police officers must be constantly alert for suspicious activity or the threat of harm, teens need to be careful not to alarm the officer by sudden movements or unpleasant words. Just in case your teen is pulled over by the police, rehearse the following with your teen:

- Pull over to the side of the road.

- Stay seated in the car with both hands on the steering wheel.

- Be polite, answering questions with respect.

- Follow directions and cooperate with police requests, such as taking breathalyzer test.

- Do not drive away until you have been given permission.

## Looking Out for Your Teen

**Health Alert**

If your teen has a substance abuse problem, get your child into therapy immediately. Deal with the situation as you would an illness, accepting the problem and putting your energy into supporting your child's recovery.

### Signs of substance abuse

Although almost any one of these signs can appear in a normal, nondrug-using teen, if you see several of these signs together, your child may have a substance abuse problem.

Call your doctor to find out how to get help if your child: spends too much time alone; stops talking or argues frequently with family members; drastically changes style of dress or hair; ignores homework and has dropping grades; drops old friends; has new friends who are less familiar and less friendly to adults; has frequent or unexplained injuries; sleeps poorly or complains of tiredness; develops irregular eating habits; has bloodshot eyes, very large or small pupils; has frequent "colds" or nosebleeds; has unusual odors on clothing; seems "jumpy" or hyperactive; has mood swings including irritability, depression, hostility, or paranoia; keeps drug paraphernalia; attempts to or runs away from home; or steals money or valuables from your home.

Remember, children need love most when they are the most unlovable.

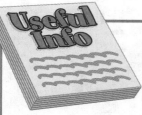

## Family Feuding

From your teen's 14th birthday through the 16th year, you can expect to have some trying times. These are the years when you are most likely to have difficulty getting along with your teen and your teen will have the most difficulty getting along with you.

Several studies have been reported about family relationships during the teen years. Compare your family's experience with the following:

- Ninety percent of 16-year-old teens report getting along well with their mother. Seventy-five percent report good relations with their dad.

- Adolescent girls report a minor conflict with parent every one-and-a-half days. Adolescent boys report a minor conflict every four days. Seventy-five percent of the conflicts are between mother and teen. Mother-daughter conflicts last an average of 15 minutes. Mother-son conflicts last an average of six minutes.

- Only 1 in 5 families reports serious difficulty with parent-child relationships.

## Late to Bed, Late to Rise

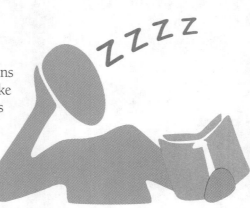

Weekend morning sleep-ins are your teen's way to make up for missed sleep. Teens need nine to 10 hours of sleep per night. Chronic daytime sleepiness, poor grades in morning classes, or drowsiness when driving are signs that your teen needs a better sleep routine every day of the week.

## Take these Signs Seriously

**Health Alert**

If your teen shows signs of serious depression, get help for your child immediately. Deal with the situation as you would an illness, accepting the problem and putting the energy into supporting your child's recovery.

### Signs of depression

Teens are often moody, dress in black day after day, and can't seem to hear anything you say. While you will learn to ignore some behaviors, other behaviors are signs of a serious problem and must not be ignored.

The following are warning signs of severe depression. Call your doctor and ask for help if your child: constantly complains of stomachaches, headaches or tiredness; sleeps too much or too little; loses or gains weight very quickly; neglects appearance; increases risky behaviors – drugs, alcohol, unsafe sex, and drinking and driving; loses interest in school and friends – falling grades, dropping out of activities, cutting classes and withdrawing from friends and family; seems suddenly cheerful after a long period of depression; makes statements like "I feel dead inside;" seems preoccupied with death in choice of music and clothing and talks frequently about friends who have died; or gives away prized possessions, writes a will, or makes other "final" arrangements.

## A Matter of Life and Death

Call a suicide crisis hotline, local emergency department, 911, or your child's doctor if your child: complains of feeling hopeless; says, "I'd be better off dead;" or has a specific plan for committing suicide. Take suicide seriously.

### *Risk factors for suicide*

Suicide is the third leading cause of death in the teen years. For every teen suicide, there are 200 suicide attempts. Risk factors include:

- previous suicide attempts
- family history of suicide
- friends who have committed suicide
- access to a gun
- history of mood, conduct, or psychotic disorders
- problems with impulse control
- concerns about sexual identity, homosexuality
- history of physical or sexual abuse
- depression

Source: *Bright Futures*, 2nd edition

## A Call to Action

The SOS (Signs of Suicide) Program trains people how to ACT if a friend or child is severely depressed and possibly suicidal. ACT stands for Acknowledge, Care and Treatment (for teenagers, the "T" stands for "Tell a responsible adult"). Call 1-800-573-4433 to locate a training site.

# Resources

## Great Book List
### Birth to 6 Months

*Goodnight Moon*
By Margaret Wise Brown and Clement Hurd

*Pat the Bunny*
By Dorothy Kunhardt

*Chicka Chicka Boom Boom*
By Bill Martin, Jr., John Archambault and Lois Ehlert

*I Love You as Much…*
By Laura Krauss Melmed and Henri Sorenson

*The Runaway Bunny*
By Margaret Wise Brown and Clement Hurd

*My First Songs*
By Jane Manning

### 6 Months to 1 Year

*Corduroy*
By Don Freeman

*The Very Hungry Caterpillar*
By Eric Carle

*Mr. Brown Can Moo, Can You?*
*Dr. Seuss's Book of Wonderful Noises*
By Dr. Seuss

*The Snowy Day*
By Ezra Jack Keats

*Curious George*
By H.A. Rey

*The Lady with the Alligator Purse*
By Nadine Bernard Westcott

## The Toddler Years: 1 and 2

*Big Red Barn*
By Margaret Wise Brown and Felicia Bond

*Cows in the Kitchen*
By June Crebbin and Katherine McEwen

*McElligot's Pool*
By Dr. Seuss

*Miss Spider's Tea Party*
By David Kirk

*Monster Munchies*
By Laura Numeroff and Nate Evans

*Papa, Please Get the Moon for Me*
By Eric Carle

## Preschool: 3 to 5

*Where the Wild Things Are*
By Maurice Sendak

*Babar Series*
By Jean DeBrunhoff

*The Napping House*
By Audrey Wood

*King Bidgood's in the Bathtub*
By Audrey Wood

*Sylvester and the Magic Pebble*
By William Steig

*Green Eggs and Ham*
By Dr. Seuss

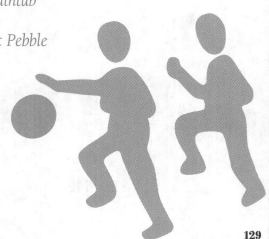

# Resources

## School Age: 6 to 11

*There's a Nightmare in my Closet*
By Mercer Mayer

*Snowflake Bentley*
By Jacqueline Briggs Martin

*Alexander and the Terrible, Horrible, No Good, Very Bad Day*
By Judith Viorst

*Charlotte's Web*
By E.B. White

*Harry Potter Series*
By J.K. Rowling

*Chronicles of Narnia*
By C.S. Lewis

## Adolescents: 12 to 21

**Middle School**

*Anne of Green Gables*
By Lucy Maud Montgomery

*A Wrinkle in Time*
By Madeline L'Engle

*David Copperfield*
By Charles Dickens

**High School**

*Tender is the Night*
By F. Scott Fitzgerald

*Brave New World*
By Aldous Huxley

*I Know Why the Caged Bird Sings*
By Maya Angelou

# Organizations
## General Growth and Development Information

*The American Academy of Pediatrics*
141 Northwest Point Boulevard
P.O. Box 747
Elk Grove Village, Illinois 60009-0747
800-433-9016 (phone)
847-228-1281 (fax)
www.aap.org

*Brilliant Beginnings, LLC*
P.O. Box 13050
Long Beach, California 90803
800-432-1357
www.brilliantbeginnings.com

*Centers for Disease Control
National AIDS Clearinghouse*
P.O. Box 6003
Rockville, Maryland 20849-6003
800-458-5231

*Children's Defense Fund*
25 E Street, N.W.
Washington, D.C. 20001
202-628-8787
www.childrensdefense.org

*National Child Care Information Center*
www.nccic.org

*Riley Hospital for Children*
702 Barnhill Drive
Indianapolis, Indiana 46202
317-274-5000
www.rileyhospital.org

# Resources

*Riley Hospital Community Education Department*
Riley Hospital for Children
575 West Drive, Room 008
Indianapolis, Indiana 46202-5272
317-274-2964
www.rileyforkids.org

## Specific Growth and Development Information

### Brain Development

*I Am Your Child Campaign*
P.O. Box 15605
Beverly Hills, California 90209
888-447-3400
www.iamyourchild.org

*Johnson and Johnson Pediatric Institute*
www.jjpi.com

*Brain Wonders*
www.zerotothree.org/brainwonders/index.html

*Zero to Three National Center for Infants, Toddlers, and Families*
2000 M Street, NW Suite 200
Washington, D.C. 20036
202-638-1144
www.zerotothree.org

*The Ounce of Prevention Fund*
www.ounceofprevention.org

# Development

*First Steps*
Indiana's Early Intervention System for Infants, Toddlers & their Families
800-441-STEP
317-232-1144
www.state.in.us/fssafirst_step
First Steps assures that all Indiana families with infants and toddlers experiencing developmental delays or disabilities have access to early intervention services close to home. Families can contact their county office for more information on eligibility and available services.

## Educational Resources

*National Association for the Education of Young Children (NAEYC)*
1509 16th Street, N.W.
Washington, D.C. 20036
800-424-2460
202-232-8777
www.naeyc.org

## Mental Health

*American Psychiatric Association*
1400 K Street, N.W.
Washington, D.C. 20005
202-682-6000

*National Institute of Mental Health*
*Public Information Office*
6001 Executive Boulevard
Bethesda, Maryland 20892-9663
301-443-4513

# Resources

## Sexuality

*Planned Parenthood Federation of America*
810 Seventh Avenue
New York, New York 10019
212-541-7800
Community resource programs and educational materials, such as brochures, videos and books, are available at various health centers located throughout the state. Call 800-421-3731, ext. 142, to find the nearest Planned Parenthood.

*Sexuality Information and Education Council of the United States*
130 West 42nd Street, #350
New York, New York 10036
212-819-9770

## Special Needs

*Camp Riley*
Riley Memorial Association
50 S. Meridian, Suite 500
Indianapolis, Indiana 46204
317-634-4474
www.rileykids.org/camp
Provides traditional camp experiences for children with disabilities.

*Indiana Parent Information Network*
1755 Kingway Drive, Suite 105
Indianapolis, Indiana 46205
317-254-8683
800-964-4746
A not-for-profit organization where parents, professionals and volunteers work together to support children with special needs.

## Substance Abuse

*Al-Anon/Alateen Family Group Headquarters*
1600 Corporate Landing Parkway
Virginia Beach, Virginia 23454
800-344-2666
757-563-1600

*National Clearinghouse for Alcohol and Drug Information*
P.O. Box 2345
Rockville, Maryland 20847-2345
800-729-6686 (phone)
301-468-6433 (fax)

*PRIDE Youth Programs*
4684 South Evergreen
Newaygo, Michigan 49337
800-668-9277 (phone)
231-652-2461 (fax)
www.prideyouthprograms.org

*Students Against Destructive Decisions (SADD)*
Formerly Students Against Driving Drunk
255 Main Street
P.O. Box 800
Marlboro, Massachusetts 01752
508-481-3568
www.saddonline.com

# Recommended Books

*Brilliant Beginnings Guidebook: Baby Birth Basics: Birth to 12 Months*
By Brilliant Beginnings, LLC (2000)

*Brilliant Beginnings Guidebook: Toddler Brain Basics: 12 to 24 Months*
By Brilliant Beginnings, LLC (2000)

*Brilliant Beginnings Guidebook: Toddler Next Steps: 24 to 36 Months*
By Brilliant Beginnings, LLC (2000)

# Resources

*The Difficult Child*
By Stanley Turecki, M.D., Bantam Books (1995)

*The Nanas and the Papas:*
*A Boomers' Guide to Grandparenting*
By Kathryn and Allan Zullo, Andrews McMeel Publishing
(1998)

*The Read-Aloud Handbook*
By Jim Trelease, Penguin Books (1995)

## Web Sites for Parents and Kids

*PBS Kids*
www.pbs.org/kids/
This Web site is great for children and adults. Kids enjoy their
favorite PBS characters while reading, playing games, and
doing other educational activities. This site also offers parents
several educational goals for children of all ages. (Ages 2-12)

*World of Discovery*
www.discovery.com
Created by the Discovery Channel, this Web site offers many
activities to share with your preschooler. (Ages 3 and up)

*The Children's Literature Web Guide*
www.Acs.ucalgary.ca/~dkbrown/index.html
This Web site for parents provides a collection of information
about children's literature. It includes information about
children's book awards, popular children's authors and
additional resources found on the Web.

# Toll-Free Help Lines

## AIDS

*Center for Disease Control AIDS Hotline*
800-342-2437

*Teen AIDS*
800-440-8336

*Teens Teaching AIDS Prevention*
800-234-8336
Monday through Thursday, 4 to 8 p.m. (CST)

## Alcohol and Drugs

*Hazelden Foundation (drug and alcohol treatment)*
800-257-7800

## Child Abuse

*Hit Home Hotline (youth crisis such as suicide, abuse, pregnancy, depression, counseling, and intervention)*
800-448-4663

*National Child Abuse Hotline*
800-422-4453

## Contraception

*Planned Parenthood*
800-230-7526

## Babysitting

*Safe Sitter National Headquarters*
5670 Caito Drive #172
Indianapolis, Indiana 46226
317-543-3840
800-255-4089
317-545-SAFE (7233) (fax)
www.safesitter.org

# Resources

## Crisis

*Adolescent Crisis and Intervention and Counseling Hotline*
800-999-9999

*Hit Home Hotline (youth crisis such as suicide, abuse, pregnancy, depression, counseling, and intervention)*
800-448-4663

*National Youth Crisis Hotline*
800-448-4663

## Depression

*National Depression Screening Day*
888-782-1000

*National Depressive and Manic Depressive Association*
800-826-3632

## Drugs and Alcohol

*Hazelden Foundation (drug and alcohol treatment)*
800-257-7800

## Sexual Identity

*Gay and Lesbian Hotline*
800-347-8336
Monday through Saturday, 6:30 to 9 p.m. (PST)

## Pregnancy

*Crisis Pregnancy Counseling Center and Adoption*
800-441-2670

*Hit Home Hotline (youth crisis such as suicide, abuse, pregnancy, depression, counseling, and intervention)*
800-448-4663

*Planned Parenthood*
800-230-7526

## Runaway

*National Runaway Hotline*
800-621-4000

*National Runaway Switchboard Hotline*
*(for parents and for runaways)*
800-621-4000

## Sexually Transmitted Infection

*Centers for Disease Control AIDS Hotline*
800-342-2437

*Sexually Transmitted Disease Hotline*
800-227-8922

*Teen AIDS*
800-440-8336

*Teens Teaching AIDS Prevention*
800-234-8336
Monday through Friday, 4 to 8 p.m. (CST)

## Suicide

*Hit Home Hotline (youth crisis such as suicide, abuse, pregnancy, depression, counseling, and intervention)*
800-448-4663

# Nutrition
## Section Three

## In this Section:

- Nutrition Basics
- Healthy Habits
- Mealtime Milestones
- Fast Food Facts
- Cholesterol and Kids
- And Much More...

Well-prepared, nutritious foods... Healthy appetites...Pleasant mealtimes together...It sounds easy, but it's not – not with working parents, weight-conscious kids, and fast food chains on every corner.

Check out what you need to know about vitamins and minerals and calcium in your teen's diet and learn a little about vegetarian nutrition. While you're at it, you'll find lots of other useful information and hard-to-find facts about child nutrition.

# Nutrition Basics

## Healthy Habits for a Lifetime

### The Right Foods

Use the Food Guide Pyramid. Eat lots from the bottom, less from the middle, and little from the top. Eat more dark-green leafy vegetables, deep-yellow vegetables, fruits, and whole grain products.

### The Right Amounts

Serve your child portions that fit the three As: age, appetite, and activity. Be sure your child gets the right amount of milk. Limit the amount of fats and sweets like butter, french fries, potato chips, soft drinks, and candy.

### Daily Exercise

Exercise as a family: bike, walk, camp, swim, play ball, visit a playground, fly a kite.

A healthy diet is easy if you eat a variety of foods within a food group, follow the suggested number of servings for each of the five major food groups, and eat portions of a reasonable size. Offering smaller portions and allowing children to ask for more satisfies hunger and does not waste food.

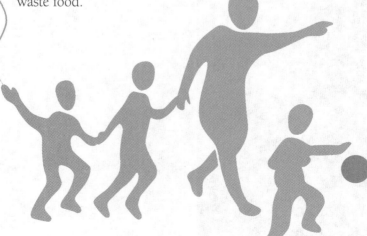

# Food Guide Pyramid

The Food Guide Pyramid is a guide to healthy food choices for good daily nutrition. The Food Guide Pyramid is based on the recommendations of the United States Department of Agriculture.

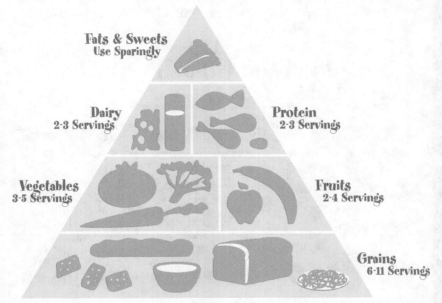

U.S. Department of Agriculture sample diets with portion size for children of various age groups can be found on the following pages.

*Dairy:* The dairy group contains foods like milk, cheese, ice cream, and yogurt. These foods are important for calcium.

*Protein:* The meat group contains foods like meat, poultry, fish, and peanut butter. These foods are important sources of protein, zinc, and iron.

*Vegetables:* The vegetable group contains foods such as carrots, squash, broccoli, and potatoes. These foods are important for vitamins, minerals, and fiber.

*Fruits:* The fruit group contains foods such as apples, bananas, pears, and strawberries. These foods are important sources of vitamins, minerals, and fiber.

*Grains:* The grain groups contains foods such as bread, cereal, rice, and pasta. These foods are important for vitamins, minerals, complex carbohydrates, and dietary fiber.

# Food Guide Pyramid

Variety is important for a healthy diet. Your child requires variety *among* food groups, such as grains, fruits, and vegetables. Your child also requires variety *within* food groups, such as apples, bananas, and pears.

## Using the Food Guide Pyramid
### Ages 2 to 3 Sample Diet

### Fruit Group
**2 servings each day**

Serving Size:
1/3 cup blueberries
5 medium strawberries
1/2 cup orange juice
1 small banana
1 small apple

### Vegetable Group
**3 servings each day**

Serving Size:
4-5 tablespoons cooked carrots, mashed or chopped
4-5 tablespoons cooked green beans, mashed or chopped
4-5 tablespoons potatoes, mashed or baked

### Grain Group
**6 servings each day**

Serving Size:
2/3 slice of bread
1/3 cup cooked oatmeal
1/3 cup cooked spaghetti
1/3 cup dry cereal
6 animal crackers

### Dairy Group
**2 servings each day**

Serving Size:
1 cup milk
1/2 cup yogurt (1/2 serving)
1 ounce processed cheese (1/2 serving)
1/2 cup pudding (1/2 serving)
1/2 cup frozen yogurt (1/2 serving)

### Protein Group
**total of 3.5 ozs. each day**

Serving Size:
1 egg (1 ounce)
1.5 ounces cooked poultry, ground or chopped (equal to three 1-inch cubes)
3 tablespoons ground meat

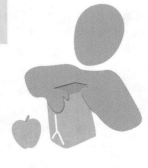

# Ages 4 to 6 Sample Diet

## Fruit Group
**2 servings each day**

Serving Size:
1/2 cup blueberries
7 medium strawberries
3/4 cup orange juice
1 medium banana
1 medium apple
1/2 cup applesauce

## Vegetable Group
**3 servings each day**

Serving Size:
2 cooked broccoli spears
7-8 raw carrot sticks
(3 inches long)
10 french fries
1/2 cup cooked lentils
1/2 cup cooked
green beans

## Grain Group
**6 servings each day**

Serving Size:
1 ounce dry cereal
1/2 cup cooked oatmeal
1 slice of bread
1/2 cup rice or pasta
2-3 graham cracker
squares

## Dairy Group
**2 servings each day**

Serving Size:
1 cup milk
1 cup yogurt
2 oz. processed cheese
1/2 cup pudding
(1/2 serving)
1/2 cup frozen yogurt
(1/2 serving)

## Protein Group
**total of 5 ozs. each day**

Serving Size:
2-3 ounces cooked lean
meat, poultry or fish
1/2 cup cooked kidney
beans, pinto or white
beans (1 ounce)
1 egg (1 ounce)
2 tablespoons peanut
butter (1 ounce)

# Ages 7 to Adult Sample Diet

## Fruit Group
**2-4 servings each day**

Serving Size:
1/2 cup blueberries
3/4 cup orange juice
1 piece of fruit
1/2 cup applesauce

## Vegetable Group
**3-5 servings each day**

Serving Size:
1/2 cup cooked vegetables
1 cup salad greens
1 medium baked potato
10 french fries

## Grain Group
**6-11 servings each day**

Serving Size:
1 slice bread
1/2 cup – 3/4 cup
dry cereal
1/2 cup rice or pasta

## Dairy Group
**2-3 servings each day**

Serving Size:
1 cup milk
1 cup yogurt
2 oz. processed cheese
1/2 cup frozen yogurt
(1/2 serving)

## Protein Group
**total of not more
than 6 ozs. each day**

Serving Size:
2-3 ounces cooked lean
meat, poultry, fish or tofu
1-2 eggs

# Before the Baby Arrives

You begin making choices about feeding your baby long before your baby is born. Pregnancy provides you with the chance to think about the food you eat, how you will feed your baby, and the eating habits you want for your growing family.

## Eating for Two

- Expect to gain 25-35 pounds.

- Practice good family mealtime habits, such as eating together with the TV off.

- Tape the Food Guide Pyramid* to your refrigerator door and use it to guide your food choices.

- Eat calcium-rich food such as dairy products, calcium-fortified orange juice, broccoli, and leafy green vegetables.

- Eat iron-rich food such as meat, poultry, fish, liver, legumes, soybean products, dried fruits, and iron-fortified cereals.

- Eat food rich in folic acid such as leafy green vegetables, fruits, milk, and folic acid-fortified cereals. Check with your doctor to be sure your folic acid intake is adequate.

- Be faithful in taking the prenatal vitamin and mineral supplement your doctor recommends.

- Avoid alcohol, caffeine, and tobacco products.

*See *Resources* pages at the end of this section for information on how to obtain a Food Guide Pyramid.

## Brain Fact

Daily folic acid intake of 600 micrograms throughout pregnancy decreases your baby's chance of a birth defect involving the baby's spine and nervous system.

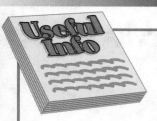

## Vitamins and Minerals

*To absorb more iron from your diet:*
Eat iron-rich food at the same sitting
with foods rich in vitamin C, such as
orange juice, tomatoes and green peppers.

*To absorb more iron from your iron supplement:* Take the iron
supplement between meals with orange juice or other juices rich
in vitamin C or with water (not with milk, coffee, or tea).

*To prevent interference with absorption of iron:* Do not take
your iron supplement at the same time you take supplementary
calcium (in doses higher than 250 milligrams) or magnesium (in
doses higher than 25 milligrams). Allow two hours between your
iron supplement and supplements of these minerals.

# Top Five Reasons to Breastfeed

1. Human breast milk is the *perfect food* for human infants and is
   superior to all commercial formulas.

2. Human breast milk composition changes from the beginning of
   the feeding to the end of the feeding, from feeding to feeding,
   and from day to day. The change in the composition of *breast
   milk makes it possible to meet your baby's changing nutritional needs.*

3. Breastfed babies have *fewer infectious illnesses* and fewer allergic
   problems in the first year of life.

4. Nursing your baby is *good for your health, too.* Breastfeeding
   mothers recover more quickly from the pregnancy, have a faster
   return to pre-pregnancy weight, have a reduced risk of
   premenopausal breast cancer, and a reduced risk of cancer of
   the ovary.

5. Breastfeeding is *convenient and saves money.* It saves you money
   since you don't have to buy expensive infant formulas. It also
   reduces health care costs in general since breastfed babies are
   healthier than formula-fed babies.

# Before the Baby Arrives

## Doctors Advise Against Breastfeeding if...

• you have AIDS or any other disease that can be passed to your baby through your breast milk.

• you take certain medications – antithyroid, anticancer – that pass into breast milk and could harm your baby.

• you have a serious health problem such as kidney failure or heart disease.

• you use drugs such as marijuana, cocaine, or methadone, or are a heavy user of alcohol.

**Health Alert**

### No Alcohol, No Tobacco

If you are pregnant or think you could be pregnant, do not drink alcoholic drinks including beer and wine.

If you are pregnant or think you could be pregnant and use tobacco products like cigarettes or chewing tobacco, stop! Your doctor can help you find a program to break the habit.

Alcohol use during pregnancy is the most frequent cause of preventable mental retardation in the United States.

Smoking during pregnancy can cause miscarriage, fetal death, premature birth, and low birth weight.

## Vitamins and Minerals

*Do formula-fed babies require vitamin supplementation?*

Formulas are supplemented with vitamins and minerals. In the first 6 months of life when infants are exclusively formula fed, they do not require supplementary vitamins and minerals. The American Academy of Pediatrics does not recommend fluoride supplementation in babies younger than 12 months of age.

*Do breastfed babies require vitamin supplementation?*

An iron supplement will be needed no later than 4 to 6 months of age. Some physicians recommend beginning iron soon after birth.

The American Academy of Pediatrics recommends vitamin D supplementation for all breastfed babies. Your doctor will prescribe vitamin D when your baby is 6 to 8 weeks of age.

In addition to vitamin D, vitamin $B_{12}$ supplements are required for babies who are nursed by mothers who follow a vegan diet (a diet that excludes all food of animal origin).

## Questions&Answers

Q: Should I offer my baby water between feedings?

A: Healthy babies do not require extra water. Formula (when properly prepared) and breast milk are adequate to meet your baby's fluid needs. Juice is not recommended in the first 6 months of life.

# Birth to 6 Months

## Not Enough Breast Milk

*Signs that baby is not getting adequate breast milk*

Call your doctor if your baby:
- does not have 6-8 wet diapers a day
- fails to nurse 8-12 times a day
- does not seem content after nursing
- acts unusually irritable or unusually drowsy
- has a weak suck, gags frequently, or has difficulty latching on

Your doctor will probably want your baby to be seen right away.

## Safe Food Handling

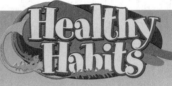

Do not save the formula (or expressed breast milk) left in the bottle after the baby has finished a feeding. Germs from your baby's mouth may have contaminated the milk, and refeeding the leftover milk may cause your baby to become ill.

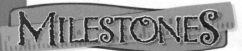

## Rice Cereal

Rice cereal is the most frequently recommended first solid food. It is usually added to the baby's diet at about 4 to 6 months.

Rice cereal is chosen because rice contains no gluten. Gluten is an allergy-triggering protein found in most other grains.

# Babies, Bottles, and Formula

**Follow directions exactly when preparing concentrated or powdered formula to ensure that the correct balance of nutrients and water is maintained.** Feeding formula that is too weak or too concentrated is dangerous to your baby's health.

**Do not use the microwave to warm your baby's bottle.** Microwaves heat unevenly, creating hot spots that can burn your baby's mouth. Microwaves may also change the composition of the milk.

**Never "prop" your baby's bottle. Babies should be held while they are feeding.** Propping is the practice of giving a baby a bottle by leaning the bottle against a pillow or other support rather than holding the baby and the bottle. Propping puts the baby at risk for choking and robs the baby of the opportunity for warm and loving interaction with the person holding the bottle.

# Questions&Answers

**Q:** Why can't babies under 1 year of age have honey?

**A:** Honey may be contaminated with the spores of the germs that cause botulism. Babies with botulism can develop muscle weakness, which sometimes progresses to paralysis and, rarely, even death.

## Child Rearing Myth

Adding rice cereal to your baby's diet will help your baby sleep through the night.

## Child Rearing Fact

Hunger is not waking your baby, and rice cereal does not help your baby sleep through the night. Your baby is a light sleeper and once awakened, can't get back to sleep without help. When your baby develops a mature sleep pattern and learns to self-comfort when awake but not hungry, you'll get a good night's sleep.

## Sample Menu for Older Infants

| FOOD | SERVING SIZE |
|---|---|
| **Breakfast** | |
| Iron-fortified cereal | 1-4 tablespoons |
| Mashed bananas[1] | 1-4 tablespoons |
| Breast milk or formula | 4-8 ounces |
| **Lunch** | |
| Ground chicken[1] | 1-2 tablespoons |
| Mashed cooked carrots[1] | 1-4 tablespoons |
| Toast with butter | 1/4-1/2 slice |
| Chopped peaches | 1-4 tablespoons |
| Breast milk or formula | 4-8 ounces |
| **Snack** | |
| Crackers | 1-2 |
| Apple juice or apple sauce[2] | 1/4-1/2 cup |
| **Dinner** | |
| Spaghetti/ground beef | 1-4 tablespoons |
| Mashed green beans[1] | 1-4 tablespoons |
| Mashed pears[1] | 1-4 tablespoons |
| Breast milk or formula | 4-8 ounces |
| **Bedtime Snack** | |
| Breast milk or formula | 6-8 ounces |

[1] Chopped can be substituted for mashed.

[2] Limit juice to 4-6 ounces per day. Offer juice in a cup, not in a bottle.

Source: U.S. Department of Agriculture

# Vitamins and Minerals

*Is fluoride supplementation needed in the first year of life?*
Fluoride is usually not needed. If your local water is not adequately fluoridated, you use a reverse osmosis filter for your drinking water, or you give your child only bottled water, your child may require fluoride supplementation in the second year of life. To check the fluoride level in your water, call your local water company. Call your county health department to have your well water tested. When you know the results, ask your child's physician if your child requires fluoride supplementation.

*Is vitamin and mineral supplementation needed for
6- to 12-month-old formula-fed babies?*
Older infants who still drink formula and who eat a variety of foods that include good sources of iron and vitamins A and C don't require supplemental vitamins. However, children with certain chronic health problems or healthy children who are finicky eaters may require vitamin and mineral supplementation.

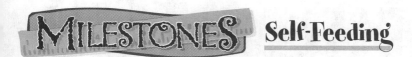 **Self-Feeding**

| Age (approximate) | Milestone |
| --- | --- |
| 5-6 months | Shows hunger or interest in food by opening mouth and leaning forward. |
| | Shows fullness or disinterest in food by turning away and leaning back. |
| 6 months | Holds own bottle. |
| 7-8 months | Self-feeds hand-held food. |
| 8-9 months | Self-feeds finger-held food. Holds cup. |
| 10-12 months | Holds spoon and aims spoon at mouth. |

## Health Alert — Food Allergies

If there is a strong history of allergy in your family, consult your physician for specific advice about feeding your infant.

As for all babies, breastfeeding is best. However, if you decide not to breastfeed, there are formulas available that are suitable.

Do not start solid foods until 6 months or later. Delay cow's milk until 1 year of age.

Source: American Academy of Pediatrics, *Guide to Your Child's Nutrition*

## Safe Food Handling — Healthy Habits

Use a clean cloth to wipe tops of baby food jars before opening jar. Do not use food from any jar if the safety button is raised, the lid does not "pop" on turning, or if the "use by" date has passed.

## Health Alert — No Bottles in Bed

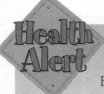

Bottles in bed increase the risk of tooth decay and ear infection.

# Home Cooking

*There are many advantages to home-prepared baby foods. They help your baby adjust to the food your family eats and are less expensive.*

Remember, when home preparing baby's food:

- Do heat, broil, steam or bake foods.

- Do use fresh vegetables within a day of purchase so that vitamin A and vitamin C are not lost. Heat vegetables in small amounts of water to preserve nutrients.

- Do cook meat to a temperature of at least 160° F (instant-read meat thermometer).

- Do use cooked food within two days.

- Don't add salt, sugar, or spices.

- Avoid using canned food with high levels of salt, sugar, or preservatives.

- Don't home prepare spinach, beets, turnips, or collard greens. These foods may contain high levels of nitrate that can cause a problem with the hemoglobin in your baby's blood.

- Don't cook acidic foods such as tomatoes in aluminum. Small amounts of aluminum may dissolve and be absorbed into the food.

- Avoid copper pots for cooking since the copper may destroy the vitamin C.

# The Toddler Years: 1 & 2

## Food Guide Pyramid
### Serving Size for a 2-Year-Old

| SERVINGS PER DAY | 1 SERVING EQUALS |
|---|---|
| **Grains[1]** | |
| 6 servings per day | 1/4-1/2 slice of bread<br>1/4 cup cereal[1], rice or pasta<br>1/4 cup dry cereal[1]<br>1-2 crackers |
| **Vegetables[2]** | |
| 3 servings per day | Cooked vegetables –<br>1 tablespoon for every year of age |
| **Fruits[3]** | |
| 2 to 3 servings per day | 1/4 cup fruit<br>1/2 piece fresh fruit<br>1/4-1/2 cup juice |
| **Dairy** | |
| 2 to 3 servings per day | 1 cup milk<br>2 ounces processed cheese<br>1-1/2 ounces natural cheese<br>1 cup yogurt |
| **Protein** | |
| 2 ounces per day | 1 ounce of solid meat<br>(two 1-inch cubes)<br>2 tablespoons of ground meat<br>2 tablespoons of cooked dry beans<br>1/2 egg, any size |

[1] Offer iron-fortified cereals (iron from cereal is well absorbed and provides 35 percent to 45 percent of the daily iron requirement).

[2] Offer rich sources of vitamin A, such as carrots, 2 to 3 times per week.

[3] Offer a rich source of vitamin C, such as 1/2 cup orange juice, every day. Limit juice to 4-6 ounces per day.

# Vitamins and Minerals

*What is the best source for vitamins and minerals for healthy toddlers?*

A well-balanced diet is the best source for vitamins and minerals for most toddlers. A healthy toddler whose diet matches the Food Guide Pyramid gets more than adequate amounts of vitamins and minerals. Even small servings of the various food groups are adequate if you pay special attention to offering good sources of iron and vitamins A and C.

*Chronic illness and vitamin and mineral supplements.*

Children who are unable to absorb nutrients from the food they eat due to gastrointestinal problems, children with food sensitivity, and children with chronic illnesses may be advised by their physician to take supplementary vitamins and minerals.

*Bright Futures: Nutrition*

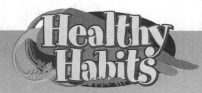

# Healthy Snacks for Older Toddlers

Offer older toddlers two or three snacks a day. Have a supply of healthy snacks available. Children should sit when eating.

**Fresh fruits:** diced apples, bananas, peaches

**Vegetables:** well-cooked and diced carrots, green beans, potatoes

**Dairy products:** sliced or diced cheese, fresh or frozen yogurt, milk

**Breads and cereals:** small pieces of pretzels or bagels

**Meats and proteins:** smooth peanut butter spread thin on bread, cracker or small strip of apple

*Bright Futures: Nutrition*

## Choking Hazards Food List

*The following foods should not be given to toddlers or children younger than age 5.*

- Hard candies, jelly beans, chewing gum
- Popcorn, raisins, marshmallows, seeds and nuts

*The following foods may be given to children between the ages of 2 and 5 only if they are cut into small pieces or strips:*

- Hot dogs (slicing lengthwise before cutting crosswise reduces the risk of choking)
- Grapes or cherries (peeling, removing seeds or pits, and cutting in half reduces the risk)
- Raw carrots, apples, celery, green beans (dicing or cutting into small strips reduces the risk)
- Peanut butter (spread thinly)
- Large chunks of any food such as meat, potatoes, or raw vegetables and fruits (dice or cut into small strips)
- Processed frozen potato products shaped like a hot dog (mash or cut length-wise)

Source: American Academy of Pediatrics, *Guide to Your Child's Nutrition*

# Questions & Answers

**Q:** How much milk should my toddler drink daily?

**A:** Two to three 6-8 ounce glasses a day is about right. Offer water when your child is thirsty. Don't overdo milk and juice between meals. Juice should be limited to 4-6 ounces per day.

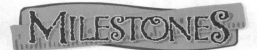 **Self-Feeding**

| Age (approximate) | Milestone |
| --- | --- |
| 18 months | Uses spoon. Holds cup with one hand. |
| 36 months | Uses spoon, fork, and gets food from plate to mouth with only occasional spills. |

## Fat in Your Toddler's Diet

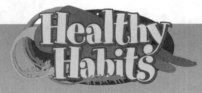

Dietary fat provides calories for growth and energy for active play. It is also important for healthy skin, shiny hair, absorbing some vitamins, and healing wounds.

Fat should supply 30 percent of your toddler's daily calories.

In the first 2 years of life, children should drink whole milk (after being weaned from breast milk or formula).

After age 2, you should gradually decrease dietary fat. Do simple things like switching from whole milk to low-fat milk and decreasing the amount of fat you cook with.

# Preschool: 3 to 5

## Food Guide Pyramid
### Serving Size for a 5-Year-Old

| SERVINGS PER DAY | 1 SERVING EQUALS |
|---|---|
| **Grains** | |
| 6 servings per day | 1 slice of bread<br>1/2 cup cooked rice or pasta<br>1 ounce dry cereal |
| **Vegetables** | |
| 3 servings per day | 1/2 cup chopped raw or cooked vegetables<br>1 cup raw leafy vegetables |
| **Fruits[1]** | |
| 2 servings per day | 1 piece of fruit<br>3/4 cup juice[1]<br>1/2 cup canned fruit |
| **Dairy** | |
| 2 servings per day | 1 cup of milk or yogurt<br>2 ounces of processed cheese<br>1-1/2 ounces natural cheese |
| **Protein** | |
| 5 ounces per day | 2 to 3 ounces of cooked lean meat, poultry, or fish<br>1/2 cup cooked dry beans<br>1 egg (counts as 1 ounce of lean meat) |

[1] Limit juice to 4-6 ounces per day.

# Vitamins and Minerals

*A well-rounded diet – not calcium supplementation – is the best source for calcium.*

Even if your child refuses to drink milk, there are plenty of other sources of dietary calcium.

| Food source | Calcium |
| --- | --- |
| Milk – 8 ounces | 300 milligrams |
| Cheddar cheese – 1 ounce | 205 milligrams |
| Calcium-fortified orange juice – 1/2 cup | 175 milligrams |
| Nonfat yogurt – 1/2 cup | 155 milligrams |
| Frozen waffle | 150 milligrams |
| Chocolate ice cream – 1/2 cup | 75 milligrams |
| Cottage cheese – 1/2 cup | 75 milligrams |
| Broccoli, steamed – 1/2 cup | 35 milligrams |

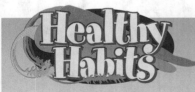

## Eating Habits

Don't allow your child to eat while watching television or playing. If your child eats while "vegging out" in front of the TV or while "surfing the Net," then eating will become a habit and not a response to hunger. Your child can take on extra calories, which add extra weight and can start a child on the "slippery slope" to obesity.

## MILESTONES

## Table Manners

At age 4, your child should be ready to learn table manners. Everyone in the family plays a part in the instruction of mealtime manners.

*Do...* sit together at the table as often as possible and include your child in the meal preparation. Do use mealtimes to discuss pleasant topics that include your child, and let your child select new foods or recipes. Always model good mealtime manners.

*Don't...* read the paper, allow toys at the table, or have the TV on. Don't give your child meal preparation jobs that are too hard or take too long. Don't argue or use mealtime for lectures or personal criticism. Don't serve large portions of new foods or expect your child to do as you say and not as you do.

*Bright Futures: Nutrition*

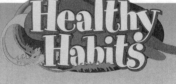

## Snacking

Use snacks to satisfy hunger, not as treats or rewards. Offer nutritious snacks 1-2 hours before meals. If meals are more than four hours apart, include some protein and fat to satisfy hungry appetites.

## Health Alert — Choking Hazards

To reduce the risk of your child choking, post a list for family, friends, and sitters of foods that are choking risks and are not to be given to your child. Insist that your child sit at the table to eat – no eating while running or playing. Don't allow tickling during mealtimes and teach your child not to talk while eating. Don't give chewing gum to a child under 6 years of age. Make sure anyone caring for your child knows what to do if your child chokes.

(See "Choking Hazards Food List" on page 158.)

# Questions & Answers

**Q:** How can I get my finicky eater to eat?

**A:** Try these ideas. Include your child in grocery shopping and food preparation. Be patient with your child and keep mealtimes pleasant. Offer nutritionally acceptable choices and role model good eating behaviors such as drinking milk at meals. Be sure to praise your child for tasting new foods. If your child refuses a new food, offer the food again in a few weeks. (Young children are discovering new foods and flavors. One study showed a new food must be offered an average of 10 times before it is accepted.)

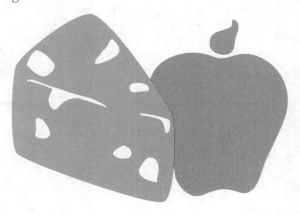

# School-Age: 6 to 11

## Food Guide Pyramid
### Serving Size for a 10-Year-Old

| SERVINGS PER DAY | 1 SERVING EQUALS |
|---|---|
| **Grains[1]** | |
| 6 to 11 servings per day | 1 slice of bread |
| | 1/2 cup cereal[1], rice or pasta |
| | 4-5 crackers |
| **Vegetables[2]** | |
| 3 to 5 servings per day | 1/2 cup cooked vegetables |
| | 1 cup salad |
| **Fruits[3]** | |
| 2 to 4 servings per day | 1/2 cup canned fruit |
| | 1 piece fresh fruit |
| | 3/4 cup fruit juice |
| **Dairy** | |
| 2 to 3 servings per day | 1 cup milk or yogurt |
| | 2 ounces processed cheese |
| | 1-1/2 ounces natural cheese |
| **Protein** | |
| 2 to 3 servings per day | 1-3 ounces of cooked lean meat, poultry, fish or tofu |
| | 1/2 cup cooked dry beans |
| | 1 or 2 eggs |

[1] Offer iron-fortified cereals (iron from cereal is well absorbed and provides 35 percent to 45 percent of the daily iron requirement).

[2] Offer rich sources of vitamin A, such as carrots, 2 to 3 times per week.

[3] Offer a rich source of vitamin C, such as 3/4 cup orange juice, every day. Limit juice to 4-6 ounces per day for age 6 and 8-12 ounces per day for ages 7-11.

# Vitamins and Minerals

*Should my school-age child take a vitamin and mineral supplement?*

Vitamin and mineral supplementation is rarely required in middle childhood. If your child is healthy and eats a reasonably balanced diet, supplementation is unnecessary. Supplementation should be considered if your child has an eating disorder, poor eating habits, or if he or she follows a restrictive or alternative diet such as a fad diet, a vegan diet (excludes all food of animal origin), or a fruitarian diet (only raw and dried fruits, seeds, sprouted seeds and grains, and nuts; no cooked foods, vegetables, or animal products).

*Is megavitamin therapy safe?*

Megavitamin therapy (extremely large vitamin doses) is unsafe. If you are tempted to try megadose vitamin therapy for your child or for yourself, beware! Vitamins or minerals in very large amounts can lead to serious health problems. Fat soluble vitamins – A, D, E, and K – are stored in the body and, if taken in large doses, can build up to toxic levels causing problems such as deafness, kidney stones, headaches, and blurred vision. When high dose vitamin or mineral supplementation is appropriate, it needs to be prescribed and monitored by a physician.

## Useful Info

## Benefits of Breakfast

Breakfast really matters. Studies show that children who don't eat breakfast have difficulty concentrating and staying alert at the beginning of the school day. Eating breakfast actually improves school performance.

## Breakfast Ideas

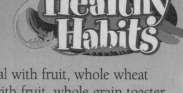

**The following foods are easy to prepare and can be eaten for breakfast:** cold cereal with fruit, whole wheat toast with peanut butter, yogurt with fruit, whole grain toaster waffles topped with fresh or canned fruits, breakfast bars with milk, and warmed up leftover pizza.

**The following foods can be eaten as a breakfast on-the-run:** granola bar with milk, bagel or toasted English muffin with peanut butter, raisin/bran or fruit/oatmeal muffin with juice, crackers and cheese with juice.

## Food Handling

**Packing school lunches:**

- Purchase an insulated, soft pack and an unbreakable thermos.
- Use plastic containers for crushable foods.
- Thoroughly wash and dry all reusable containers.
- Wash hands before preparing food.
- Choose foods that require no refrigeration.
- Wash fruit before packing.
- Peel and wash vegetables before packing.
- Pack portions that match your child's appetite.

# Questions&Answers

**Q:** What are some good sources of fiber for my child's school lunch box?

**A:** Sandwiches made with whole wheat bread provide a good source of fiber. Fresh fruits and vegetables such as apples, celery, and carrots are all high fiber foods that are safe bets as child pleasers.

## Choosing Good Nutrition at the Vending Machine

| *Leave the…* | *Instead, choose…* |
| --- | --- |
| potato chips | baked tortilla chips |
| cheese snacks | pretzels, popcorn |
| candy bars | granola bar, trail mix |
| soft drinks | water, low-fat milk or chocolate milk |
| ice cream | pure fruit popsicle, frozen yogurt |
| cookies | graham crackers, fig bars |

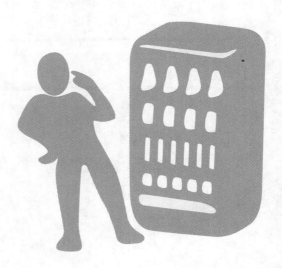

## Food Guide Pyramid
### Serving Size for Teens

| SERVINGS PER DAY | 1 SERVING EQUALS |
|---|---|
| **Grains[1]** | |
| 6 to 11 servings per day | 1 slice of bread |
| | 3/4 cup dry cereal[1] |
| | 1/2 cup cooked cereal |
| | 1/2 cup cooked pasta or rice |
| **Vegetables[2]** | |
| 3 to 5 servings per day | 1/2 cup cooked vegetables |
| **Fruits[3]** | |
| 2 to 4 servings per day | 1 medium piece fresh fruit |
| **Dairy** | |
| 2 to 4 servings per day | 1 cup milk or yogurt |
| | 1-1/2 ounces natural cheese |
| | 2 ounces processed cheese |
| | (1-1/2-inch cube or 2 precut slices) |
| **Protein** | |
| 2 to 3 servings per day | 2-3 ounces cooked, lean meat, |
| | poultry, fish or tofu |

[1] Offer iron-fortified cereals (iron from cereal is well absorbed and provides 35 percent to 45 percent of the daily iron requirement).

[2] Offer rich sources of vitamin A, such as carrots, 2 to 3 times per week.

[3] Offer a rich source of vitamin C, such as 3/4 cup orange juice, every day. Limit juice to 8-12 ounces per day.

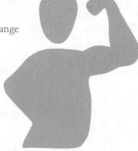

## Medications and Mealtime

Check the patient information sheet enclosed with medications for directions about the timing of the medication in relation to foods and/or drinks and any food or drinks to avoid when taking the medication.

# Vitamins and Minerals

*Do any of the medications commonly prescribed for teenagers interact with vitamins?*

Several medications commonly prescribed for teens, like oral contraceptives, certain antibiotics, and the acne medicine *Accutane* change the requirement for specific vitamins or minerals. Ask your child's doctor for specific directions.

*Does my teenager need a calcium supplement?*

Some teens may need calcium supplements. Four servings of milk and dairy products provide adequate calcium to meet daily recommendations. Teens who avoid dairy products need to increase their intake of other foods high in calcium, such as calcium-fortified orange juice. For teens with inadequate dietary calcium intake, many doctors suggest taking a nonprescription calcium-containing antacid tablet or a soft chewable calcium supplement daily.

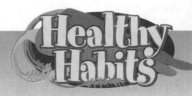

## Food Supplements are Second Choice

Spend your money on good foods not on food supplements. Problems with absorption, inferior quality, and missing nutrients make supplements second choice.

# Adolescents: 12 to 21

## Calorie and Nutrient Requirements for Teens

### Recommended Dietary Allowances

| | CALORIES | PROTEIN (g) | IRON (mg) | ZINC (mg) | CALCIUM (mg) |
|---|---|---|---|---|---|
| **Males 11-14** | 2500 | 45 | 12 | 15 | 1300 |
| **Males 15-18** | 3000 | 59 | 12 | 15 | 1300 |
| **Males 19-24** | 2900 | 58 | 10 | 15 | 1000 |
| **Females 11-14** | 2200 | 46 | 15 | 12 | 1300 |
| **Females 15-18** | 2200 | 44 | 15 | 12 | 1300 |
| **Females 19-24** | 2200 | 46 | 15 | 12 | 1000 |

Note: g=grams; mg=milligrams
Source: National Academy of Science

## Nutrition in the Fast Lane

| | CALORIES | PROTEIN (g) | FAT (g) | SODIUM (mg) |
|---|---|---|---|---|
| **Kentucky Fried Chicken Drumstick & Wing** | 390 | 29 | 27 | 1169 |
| **McDonald's Big Mac** | 590 | 24 | 34 | 1090 |
| **McDonald's Large Fry** | 540 | 8 | 26 | 350 |
| **Pizza Hut 2 Slices Cheese** | 480 | 12 | 20 | 1300 |
| **Subway 6" Veggie Delite** | 200 | 7 | 23 | 500 |

Note: g=grams; mg=milligrams

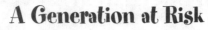

# A Generation at Risk

Soft drinks have replaced milk as the mealtime drink of teenagers.

When teens drink a 12-ounce can of cola instead of a 12-ounce glass of milk, they lose 450 milligrams of calcium, which is 1/3 of their daily requirement of calcium.

Only 1 in 5 teen girls gets the recommended daily amount of calcium.

The recommended daily amount of calcium is critical to build strong bones.

Calcium can be lost from bone throughout life, but it can only be added during adolescence and through the 20s.

Inadequate calcium intake in teen years means an increased risk of osteoporosis and hip fractures in older adults.

# Calories to Grow On

Teens who restrict the number of calories they eat may be stunting their growth. When calories are limited, growth takes a back seat. Calories go first to provide the energy for basic life processes. Next, they provide fuel for physical activity. If there are calories left over, they are used for growth. When there are no extra calories, the teen's growth suffers. Inadequate calorie intake can also affect emotions and the body's ability to fight infection.

# Adolescents: 12 to 21

Nutrition

## The Iron Age

Teens require iron – almost half again as much as needed during the preteen years.

Boys require the extra iron to keep up with the demands of new muscles and more blood for a bigger body. Girls require the extra iron for growth and to replace the iron lost in menstrual blood.

Iron requirements are further increased for males and females who are active in athletics.

## Strong Bones by the Glass

| DRINK (8 fluid ounces) | CALORIES | CALCIUM (mg) |
|---|---|---|
| 2% Milk | 121 | 300 |
| Skim Milk | 86 | 300 |
| Low-fat Chocolate Milk | 190 | 300 |
| Calcium-fortified Orange Juice | 110 | 350 |
| Chocolate Shake | 300 | 250 |

Note: mg=milligrams

## Empty Calories that Leave Holes

| DRINK (8 fluid ounces) | CALORIES | CALCIUM (mg) |
|---|---|---|
| Coke | 97 | 9 |
| Diet Coke | 0 | 12 |
| Sweetened Iced Tea | 80 | 8 |
| Lemonade | 110 | 8 |

Note: mg=milligrams

172

# Fat in Your Child's Diet

## The Skinny on Fat

*Birth to 2*

- To assure proper growth and brain development, half of your child's daily calories should come from fat.

*2 to 18*

- Fat should supply 30 percent of your child's daily calories.

- Reduce saturated fats to no more than 10 percent of the day's calories. Foods high in saturated fat include butter, lunch meats, and bacon.

- Limit cholesterol in the diet to less than 300 milligrams daily. Foods high in cholesterol include eggs, processed cheese, and shrimp.

- Check food labels for nutritional information including cholesterol and saturated fat content.

---

## Cholesterol Screening

The American Academy of Pediatrics recommends testing for a child:

- whose parents or grandparents have had a heart attack or have been diagnosed with blocked arteries or have a disease affecting the blood vessels (such as a stroke) before age 55.

- whose parents have a high blood cholesterol (200 mg/dl or higher).

- who is adopted or whose family medical history is unknown.

- who has other risk factors likely to cause early onset of coronary heart disease, such as cigarette smoking, severe obesity, diabetes, or high blood pressure.

Note: mg/dl=milligrams per 100 milliliters

# Fat in Your Child's Diet

## Cholesterol Profile in Children and Adolescents

| CLASSIFICATION | TOTAL CHOLESTEROL* | LOW-DENSITY LIPOPROTEIN (LDL)* |
|---|---|---|
| **Acceptable** | less than 170 | less than 110 |
| **Borderline** | 170-199 | 110-129 |
| **High** | more than 200 | more than 130 |

*mg/dl=milligrams per 100 milliliters
Source: American Academy of Pediatrics

# Understanding Test Results

A cholesterol profile measures the level of fats in the blood – both harmful fats and helpful ones. The two types of cholesterol most commonly measured are the high-density lipoprotein (HDL), which is the "good" cholesterol, and the low-density lipoprotein (LDL), which is the "bad" cholesterol. The LDL cholesterol contributes to the build-up of problem-causing fat deposits along blood vessel walls.

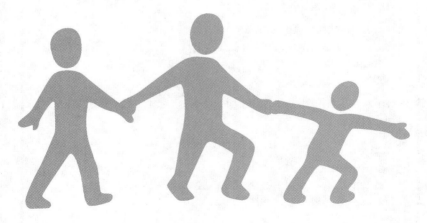

# Vegetarian Diets

## Vegetarian Diets and Health

"Vegetarian diets are healthful and nutritionally adequate when appropriately planned. Both vegetarian and nonvegetarian diets have the potential to be either beneficial or detrimental to health."

– American Dietetic Association Policy Statement, 1988.

## Attention Parents of Vegetarians
### What Parents Should Know about Vegetarian Diets

"I've decided not to eat meat anymore." "No meat for me." As increasing numbers of teens make the decision to pass up the traditional "meat and potatoes" diet of the Midwest, more and more parents are facing mealtime and nutritional challenges that can prove quite frustrating. Though it may be tempting, frustrated parents must not throw up their hands and abandon the role of nutritional "watchdog." A vegetarian diet can be a healthy diet, but only when the correct foods in the correct combinations are eaten on a regular basis.

Vegetarian means different things to different teens. Begin by finding out what being a vegetarian means to your child. Use the chart on the next page to determine what type of vegetarian your child is.

## Bright is Right

### Healthy Habits

When it comes to choosing vegetables and fruits, bright is right. Brightly colored vegetables and fruits such as spinach, kale, strawberries, and blueberries have high concentrations of nutrients called phytochemicals. Phytochemicals protect against cancer and cardiovascular disease and promote good health.

# Vegetarian Diets

## Vegetarian Variations

**To use this chart:** Find the food groups that your child regularly includes in his or her diet. The categories with "✔" pictured indicate that these foods are eaten. The "✘" indicate that foods in this group are not eaten. When you find the line that best matches the food groups your child eats, the "Type of Vegetarian" column tells you the official name for that diet. A diet that includes eggs and dairy products (lacto-ovo vegetarian) is the most common vegetarian diet and the least risky for nutritional problems. Note: A diet that includes seafood and poultry (partial vegetarian) is not truly vegetarian.

| TYPE OF VEGETARIAN | GRAINS, FRUITS & VEGETABLES | DAIRY PRODUCTS | EGGS | SEAFOOD | POULTRY | MEAT |
|---|---|---|---|---|---|---|
| Partial Vegetarian | ✔ | ✔ | ✔ | ✔ | ✔ | ✘ |
| Lacto-ovo Vegetarian | ✔ | ✔ | ✔ | ✘ | ✘ | ✘ |
| Lacto Vegetarian | ✔ | ✔ | ✘ | ✘ | ✘ | ✘ |
| Ovo-Vegetarian | ✔ | ✘ | ✔ | ✘ | ✘ | ✘ |
| Vegan | ✔ | ✘ | ✘ | ✘ | ✘ | ✘ |

## Health Benefits

A well-planned vegetarian diet offers the following health benefits:

- A low rate of obesity because plant foods contain fewer calories.
- A low rate of heart disease due to the low cholesterol level and low saturated fat level in plant food.
- A low rate of certain cancers due to the protection provided by antioxidants naturally found at high levels in some plants.
- A low rate of diabetes and gall bladder disease.
- The advantage of a diet that is naturally high in fiber.

## Health Alert

### A Note to Vegetarians

*To avoid serious nutritional deficiencies with vegetarian or alternative diets, you should seek advice from your physician or a registered dietitian.*

An unplanned vegetarian diet (especially one that does not include eggs or dairy products) increases the chances of:

- Calorie deficiency, since plant foods are so bulky that appetites may be gone before adequate calories are eaten.
- Protein deficiency, since plant proteins are less complete and less well used by the body (see "Complete proteins – Vegetarian style").
- Vitamin $B_{12}$ deficiency, since vitamin $B_{12}$ can only be absorbed from animal products.
- Vitamin D deficiency, since vitamin D is found in egg yolks, fish liver oil, and vitamin D-fortified milk and butter.
- Calcium deficiency, since the best sources of calcium are milk and milk products.
- Zinc and iron deficiency, since meat and poultry are the richest source of zinc and iron.

# Vegetable Protein vs. Animal Protein

Protein is an essential nutrient needed by every cell in the body. Amino acids are the building blocks of protein. Certain amino acids (essential amino acids) must be supplied by the diet. Complete proteins contain all of the essential amino acids. Most animal proteins are complete and most vegetable proteins are incomplete. Vegetable proteins can be combined in several ways to create complete proteins. Vegetable protein can also meet nutritional requirements when combined with the complete protein from small amounts of eggs and dairy products. (See "Complete proteins – Vegetarian style.")

# Vegetarian Diets

## Mix and Match Amino Acids for Complete Protein

To form a complete protein, mix and match foods so that the amino acid strength of one food balances the weakness of the other. (See "Complete proteins – Vegetarian Style" below.)

|  | GOOD SOURCE FOR THESE AMINO ACIDS | POOR SOURCE FOR THESE AMINO ACIDS |
|---|---|---|
| **Legumes** (soybeans, lentils, peas, black-eyed peas, chickpeas, peanuts) | Lysine, Isoleucine | Tryptophan, Methionine, Cystine |
| **Grains** (rice, wheat, oats, corn, barley, rye, buckwheat) | Tryptophan, Methionine, Cystine | Lysine, Isoleucine |
| **Seeds and Nuts** (sesame, sunflower, pine nuts, pecans) | Tryptophan, Methionine, Cystine | Lysine, Isoleucine |
| **Other Vegetables** (potatoes, eggplant, spinach, sweet potatoes, broccoli, green peas) | Tryptophan, Lysine | Isoleucine, Methionine, Cystine |
| **Eggs** | All | None |
| **Milk Products** | All | None |

## Complete Proteins - Vegetarian Style

### Grains with Legumes
Rice and black-eyed peas
Peanut butter sandwiches
Bean taco

### Grains with Milk
Oatmeal with milk
Macaroni and cheese
Pizza

### Legumes with Seeds
Hummus (chickpea and sesame paste)

### Grains with Eggs
Rice pudding
French toast
Egg salad sandwich

### Other Vegetables with Milk and Eggs
Eggplant parmesan
Vegetable omelet
Vegetable quiche

# Dietary Reference

## FOOD SOURCES FOR VITAMINS AND MINERALS

| | |
|---|---|
| **Vitamin A** | milk, butter, carrots*, liver, eggs, fruit, dark green and yellow vegetables |
| **Vitamin $B_6$** | chicken, fish, liver, cereals, bread, spinach, green beans, bananas, peanuts* |
| **Vitamin $B_{12}$** | only in animal foods, meat, fish, eggs, milk |
| **Vitamin C** | citrus fruits, cantaloupe, berries, green peppers, tomatoes, dark green vegetables, potatoes |
| **Vitamin D** | fortified milk, liver, eggs, salmon and other fish |
| **Vitamin E** | vegetable oils, seeds*, nuts*, soybeans, wheat germ, green leafy vegetables, whole-grain cereals |
| **Vitamin K** | green leafy vegetables, peas, potatoes, liver, milk, dairy products |
| **Folic acid** | orange juice, asparagus, broccoli, spinach, lima beans, green leafy vegetables, other citrus fruits, milk, whole grain products |
| **Calcium** | milk, cheese, yogurt, calcium-fortified orange juice, green leafy vegetables, clams |
| **Phosphorus** | milk, meat, poultry, fish, eggs, dried beans, peas |
| **Magnesium** | green leafy vegetables, nuts*, soybeans, seeds*, whole grains and cereals |
| **Iron** | liver, meat, egg yolk, green vegetables, whole grains (especially iron-fortified cereals), legumes, nuts* |
| **Zinc** | meat, liver, eggs, poultry, seafood |

*Choking hazard for child under 5 years of age.

# Resources

*Parents: To get a Food Guide Pyramid, contact the U.S. Department of Agriculture Center for Nutrition and Policy and Promotion (listing is on next page).*

## Organizations
### General Nutrition Information

*The American Academy of Pediatrics*
141 Northwest Point Boulevard
P.O. Box 747
Elk Grove Village, Illinois 60009-0747
800-433-9016 (phone)
847-228-1281 (fax)
www.aap.org

*The American Dietetic Association*
216 W. Jackson Boulevard, Suite 800
Chicago, Illinois 60606-6995
800-877-1600 (phone)
312-899-0040 (phone)
www.eatright.org

*The American Dietetic Association Hotline*
800-366-1655 (for nutritional information)

*American School Health Association*
*Food and Nutrition Council*
7263 State Route 43
P.O. Box 708
Kent, Ohio 44240-0708
330-678-1601 (phone)
330-678-4526 (fax)

*Bright Futures Project*
*National Center for Education in Maternal*
*and Child Health*
Georgetown University
2000 15th Street, North, Suite 701
Arlington, Virginia 22201-2617
703-524-7802 (phone)
703-524-9335 (fax)
www.brightfutures.org

*Food and Drug Administration Office of*
*Food Nutritional Products Labeling and Dietary Supplements*
200 C Street, S.W., Suite 1832
Washington, D.C. 20204
202-205-4561 (phone)
202-205-4594 (fax)
www.fda.gov

*Food and Nutrition Board*
*Institute of Medicine*
2101 Constitution Avenue, N.W.
Washington, D.C. 20418
202-334-1732 (phone)
202-334-2316 (fax)

*International Food Information Council*
1100 Connecticut Avenue, N.W.
Suite 430
Washington, D.C. 20036
202-296-6540 (phone)
202-296-6547 (fax)

*U.S. Department of Agriculture*
*Center for Nutrition and Policy Promotion*
3101 Park Center Drive
Room 1034
Alexandria, Virginia 22302
703-605-4266 (phone)
703-605-0809 (fax)
703-305-2167 (to order Food Guide Pyramid)

# Resources

## Specific Nutrition Issues and Concerns

### Breastfeeding

*The Academy of Breastfeeding Medicine*
P.O. Box 81323
San Diego, California 92138-1323
877-836-9947 (phone)
619-295-0058 (fax)
www.bfmed.org

*Best Start*
4809 E. Busch Boulevard
Suite 104
Tampa, Florida 33617
800-277-4975 (phone)
813-971-2280 (fax)

*La Leche League International*
1400 N. Meacham Road
Schaumburg, Illinois 60173-4048
800-525-3243 (phone)
847-519-0035 (fax)
www.lalecheleague.org

### Food Allergies

*Food Allergy Network*
10400 Eaton Place, Suite 107
Fairfax, Virginia 22030-2208
703-691-3179 (phone)
703-691-2713 (fax)
www.foodallergy.org

## Vegetarian Nutrition

*The Vegetarian Resource Group*
P.O. Box 1463
Baltimore, Maryland 21203
410-366-8343 (phone)
410-366-8804 (fax)
www.vrg.org

# Recommended Books

*Being Vegetarian*
By the American Dietetic Association, 800-877-1600

*The College Student's Guide to Eating Well on Campus*
By Ann Selkowitz Litt (2000). Tulip Hill Press

*Feed Your Child Right from Birth Through Teens*
By Albert C. Goldberg (2000). M. Evans and Co., Inc.

*The Vegetarian Way*
By Virginia Messina and Mark Messina (1996).
Crown Trade Paperbacks

*The Family Nutrition Book*
By William Sears, M.D., and Martha Sears, R.N. (1999).
Little Brown & Co.

# Web Sites for Parents and Kids

*Nutrition Café*
www.exhibits.pacsci.org/nutrition/default.html
Nutrition Café is one of the best sites on the Web for nutrition
information. It has a few games that are fun and full of information.
(Ages 5-10)

*Dole 5-a-day*
www.dole5aday.com
Created by Dole, a fruit and vegetable company, this Web site
introduces several playful characters, such as Barney Broccoli and
Bobby Banana, to help kids learn about healthy foods. (Ages 6-8)

# Resources

## Kids Food

www.kidsfood.org

This interactive site provides nutrition information for children, parents and teachers. Kids can enjoy the fun and interactive quizzes and games, while adults can learn about activities to do with their children to help them eat well and stay healthy. This site also offers a great list of books about nutrition for children. (Ages 10 and up)

## Nutrition Camp

www.nutritioncamp.com

This Web site, sponsored by Kellogg, contains basic nutrition information. It features games that test nutrition knowledge, stories about the benefits of breakfast, and a question-and-answer section. (Ages 5-10)

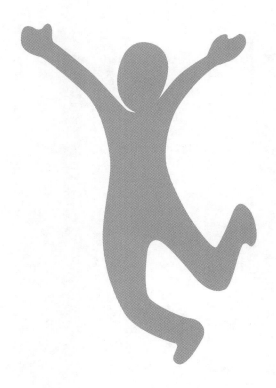

# Child Safety
## Section Four

## In this Section:

- Safety Basics
- Safety Aids
- Safety Sense
- Safety Games
- Home Fire Drills
- And Much More...

Did you know that the number of children in the United States who suffer injuries from motor vehicles in one year equals the entire population of Vincennes, Indiana? Or that the number of children injured on bicycles in one year equals the combined populations of South Bend, Anderson, Bloomington, and Evansville?

The numbers tell the story. Too many children suffer too many injuries – injuries that could be prevented.

In the *Child Safety* section, you'll discover the steps you can take to protect your child from common childhood injuries and lots of other useful information and hard-to-find facts about child safety.

Smoke alarms and safety gates are two safety aids that you already know about, but there are lots more. The Consumer Product Safety Commission rates the following safety aids as the top 12. These devices can be purchased at hardware stores, supermarkets, drug stores, and wherever baby equipment and housewares are sold. Caution: Safety devices work only if they are kept in good working order (proper installation, changing batteries at least once a year) and used as intended (consistent cooperation of older children and adults in the family).

*No safety aid replaces parental supervision.*

# Top 12 Child Safety Aids

1. *Smoke detectors.* (less than $10) Use smoke detectors on every level of your home and outside of bedrooms. Check battery monthly and change battery once a year.

2. *Carbon monoxide detectors.* ($30-$70) Use carbon monoxide detector outside bedrooms, in homes with gas or oil heat and garages that are attached.

3. *Anti-scald aids.* ($6-$30) Use anti-scald devices on faucets and showerheads to regulate water temperature. Also, if possible, set water heater temperature to 120° F.

4. *Window blind safety tassels.* (Get free window blind safety tassels by calling 1-800-506-4636.) Looped cords on window blinds are a strangulation risk for children. By cutting the loop and placing safety tassels on each cord end, the danger is removed. Ask about safety features when buying new miniblinds, vertical blinds, and draperies. With older blinds and drapery cords, hold cords tight with tension or a tie-down device.

5. *Safety gates.* ($13-$40) Use safety gates to block stairs and off-limit rooms. Purchase gates that are easy to use and that stay in place. Use screws to fasten gates to wall at tops of stairs.

6. *Outlet covers and outlet plates.* (less than $2) Buy outlet covers that are large enough to prevent choking and difficult for a child to remove.

7. *Window guards and safety netting.* ($8-$16) Use window guards and safety netting for windows, balconies, decks, and landings. Bars on window guard should be no more than 4 inches apart. Reserve at least one window in each room as fire exit.

8. *Safety latches and locks.* (less than $2) Use safety latches and locks on cabinets and drawers in kitchens, bathrooms and other areas where dangerous objects are stored. Purchase safety latches and locks that are easy to install and easy to use. They must be sturdy enough to keep children out of cabinets and drawers.

9. *Corner and edge bumpers.* ($1 and up) Purchase bumpers that stay securely on furniture. Use bumpers to soften falls against sharp or rough edges.

10. *Door knob covers and door locks.* (cover: $1; lock: $5 and up) Doorknob covers keep kids out of rooms with danger. Purchase covers that work for children but can be opened quickly by an adult. Door locks should be placed high on the door, out of children's reach.

11. *Door stops and door holders.* (less than $4) Use doorstops and door holders to prevent crush injuries from doors or door hinges.

12. *Cordless phone.* ($30 and up) Useful to call for help without having to leave children.

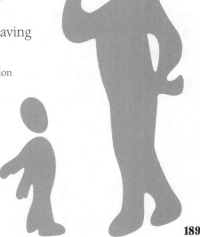

Source: U.S. Consumer Product Safety Commission

# A Letter to Parents...

*On the day your local newspaper lists the birth of your child, you probably buy a paper or get one from a friend and clip out the official announcement to put in your family record. Very likely, the newspaper list includes the names of other parents whose babies were born on the same day. Although you don't yet realize it, you will very likely have more in common with these parents than children who share the same birthday. You will share many of the same hopes and fears for your children.*

*As parents, we tend to behave in fairly predictable ways. The birth of a child (and the pregnancy) affects most of us with joy, awe, and a little bit of fear – fear that we might not be up to the job of parenting with all of its responsibilities: keeping the child healthy, protecting the child from harm, and helping the child grow and develop into a contributing member of society. It's a big job.*

*As a new parent, you are already thinking about your child's safety. Your baby, like the other babies discharged on the same day, has a safe ride home in a rear-facing child safety seat secured in the back seat of your car. Like other new parents, you have been making your home safe for your child – bumper pads in the crib, nursery monitors, and more. You are already investing time and money in the important responsibility of keeping your child safe.*

*Time passes. Safety gates and nursery monitors no longer do the job of protecting your child from danger. There are different dangers now. Your child is about to leave your safe home for the first day of school. You face the reality that your role in keeping your child safe is* decreasing, and your child's role is increasing. Your child must know how to handle dangerous situations without you. You have been preparing for this day. Very likely, your child can give his or her name and address and knows to look left-right-left before crossing the street. You have been teaching your child how to stay safe in the world.

Ten years pass and your baby-turned-teenager is preparing to drive off in the family car for the first time. Your heart skips a beat and your stomach aches with a dull, heavy pain. You taught your child safety habits. Your child can handle the car, but what about those other new drivers? What about drivers who are drinking? What if it rains? Once again, you think about what you can do to keep your child safe. You've made your home safe for your child. You've made your child safe for the world. But now that you realize all of the risks "out there," you know you haven't done enough. You want to make the world safe for your child.

There are other parents "out there" who share your concerns – parents who used child safety seats and safety gates and who taught their children how to cross the street safely. You've talked with them at back-to-school night, football games, and school fund raisers. They worry about the same problems you do – drugs, gangs, crime. These aren't problems that can be fixed easily, but they are problems that concerned parents can work on together. Join with these parents to tackle the problems in your community that threaten the safety of children.

All kids are our kids. Keeping your child safe can only be accomplished in a community where all children are safe. Your commitment to do all that you can to make your community safe for your child becomes your obligation to do all that you can to make your community safe for all children.

# Safety Basics

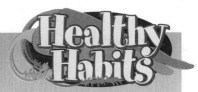

## Childhood is Risky Business

The years of first steps, birthday bikes, swimming lessons, and after-school soccer are also the years of bumps, bruises, broken bones and worse. Children are at special risk for injury for many reasons. They don't recognize danger. They are naturally curious. They are less likely to have the skills to escape from dangerous situations. Their bodies are fragile and more likely to be seriously injured. And, they depend on the safety habits of those who care for them.

## The Size of the Problem Nationwide

- Unintentional injury-related death is the leading cause of death among children 14 and under.

- In 1997, more than 6,000 children died from unintentional injuries and more than 120,000 children were permanently disabled. Almost half of the deaths from unintentional injury occur in children ages 4 and younger.

- Each year more than 14 million children ages 14 or under are treated for unintentional injuries.

- Children living in rural areas are at greater risk of serious injury resulting in death than children living in urban areas. About 150,000 children ages 14 and under suffer farm-related injuries each year.

- Most childhood injuries occur between May and August. The majority of serious injuries resulting in death occur in the evening hours.

- It is estimated that as many as 90 percent of unintentional injuries can be prevented.

Source: National SAFE KIDS Campaign

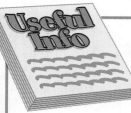

## Injuries are Not Accidents

Accidents happen by chance. They can't be predicted. They can't be prevented.

Injuries are not accidents. They *can* be predicted. They *can* be prevented.

Knowing and using good safety habits can prevent most unintentional injuries.

# Cause of Death from Unintentional Injury in Children Ages 1-14

| Rank | Cause | Percent of deaths |
|------|-------|-------------------|
| #1 | Motor vehicle | 31 |
| #2 | Drowning | 17 |
| #3 | Pedestrian | 14 |
| #4 | Fire/burn | 12 |
| #5 | Suffocation and choking | 11 |
| #6 | Bicycle | 4 |

Source: National SAFE KIDS Campaign

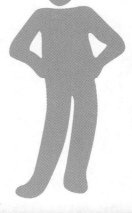

Get into the helmet habit. All bikers should wear helmets on all bike rides. Moms and dads should wear helmets. Kids on tricycles should wear helmets. Even if the bike ride is just down the driveway, your child should wear a helmet. Be consistent. Don't allow your child to ride without a helmet. Decorating a helmet with decals may make it easier to get your child's cooperation. No helmet – no bike. Get into the helmet habit. No exceptions! No excuses! No regrets!

## The Size of the Problem Nationwide

- In 1998, more than 200 children ages 14 and under died in bicycle-related crashes and more than 350,000 children age 14 and under were injured.
- Motor vehicles are involved in 90 percent of all bicycle-related deaths and 10 percent of all bicycle-related injuries.
- Nearly 60 percent of bicycle-related deaths occur on minor roads, usually within one mile of home. Bicycle injuries are four times more common in non-daylight hours.
- Bicycle helmets reduce the risk of head injury by 85 percent. It is estimated that 75 percent of bicycle-related deaths among children could be prevented by proper use of a bicycle helmet.

Source: National SAFE KIDS Campaign

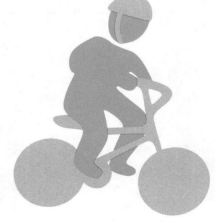

# Biking Safely

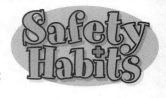

*Restrict biking to sidewalks or bike paths until age 10 or until your child demonstrates the skill and judgement to be safe in traffic.*

To protect your child from injuries, be sure your child:

- wears a bike helmet approved by the CPSC. Helmets made before March 1999 must be approved by either Snell, ANSI or ASTM and will only be available until March 2002.*

- has a helmet that fits snugly, covers the top part of the forehead and does not slide.

- has a bike that is the right size, in good repair, and is equipped with a light or front reflector, rear reflector and horn.

- knows and uses hand signals for turning left and right and stopping.

- rides on the right side of the road, with traffic.

- obeys traffic signs and signals and knows to stop and look left-right-left before entering an intersection or street, whether or not there is a stop sign.

- wears brightly colored clothing, has shoelaces securely tied, and avoids clothing that could get caught in bike wheels.

- does not ride at night or in bad weather.

- never bikes while wearing headphones.

- never rides double.

- always has at least one hand on the handlebars.

Source: American Academy of Pediatrics and National SAFE KIDS Campaign

*CPSC (Consumer Product Safety Commission), Snell (Snell Memorial Foundation), ANSI (American National Standards Institute), ASTM (American Society for Testing and Materials)

## Bicycle Safety and the Child with Special Needs

If your child is not able to use a conventional bike, the Community Education Department at Riley Hospital for Children would be glad to provide you with information about adapted bikes. For more information, visit the Professional's Area under Safety Smart at *www.rileyforkids.org* or call 317-274-2964.

# Choking

Normally when eating or drinking, food or fluid is taken into the front of the mouth, moved to the back of the mouth by the tongue, and then is swallowed into the tube leading to the stomach (esophagus). If the fluid or food (or foreign object) enters the airway instead, the person coughs or gags. There are four possibilities for what happens next. 1.) Coughing brings the food (object) out of the airway and into the back of the mouth where it is successfully swallowed. 2.) The food (object) is coughed or vomited out of the mouth. 3.) The food (object) is coughed out of the airway, then swallowed and becomes caught in the tube leading to the stomach. 4.) The food (object) is inhaled deeper into the airway, making it difficult or impossible to breathe. Difficulty breathing is a life-threatening emergency. Without immediate first aid to clear the airway, the choking victim will die.

## The Size of the Problem Nationwide

- In 1997, almost 200 children ages 14 and under died from choking. Eighty percent of these deaths occurred in children ages 4 and under.

- In 1998, 10 children died from choking on a toy or toy part. Balloons caused half of these deaths.

- Every year, approximately 5,000 children ages 14 and under receive emergency care because of an inhaled or swallowed toy or toy part.

- Food items are involved in the majority of childhood choking injuries and deaths.

- Balloon-related deaths are a risk for children ages 3 and older as well as younger children.

Source: National SAFE KIDS Campaign

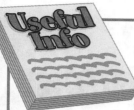

# Choking Hazard Labels

The Consumer Product Safety Commission protects children from choking as follows:

*Children under age 3:* The packaging of toys with small parts and loose pieces must display a choking hazard label with the following warning: "Choking hazard. Small parts. Not for children under 3 years."

*Children ages 3 to 6:* The packaging of toys with small parts and loose pieces must display a choking hazard label that warns parents that the toy is a choking risk.

*Children under age 8:* The packaging for balloons must display a choking hazard label that cautions: "Choking hazard. Children under 8 years can choke or suffocate on uninflated or broken balloons. Adult supervision required."

Source: National SAFE KIDS Campaign

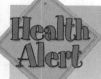

# Choking Risks and Your Child with Special Needs

If your child with special needs has difficulty swallowing, use extra care with feeding and food preparation. Children who continue to "mouth" objects are also at increased risk for choking. All caregivers must be especially careful.

# Choking

## Be Ready to Rescue

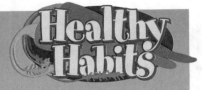

Be ready for an emergency. You and anyone who cares for your child should be trained in CPR (cardiopulmonary resuscitation). You should also be trained in CPR for infants.

Local hospitals and fire departments offer first-aid and CPR courses approved by the American Heart Association.

Written instructions for CPR and first aid should be immediately available in case of an emergency. Get several copies of CPR and first-aid instructions and place one in your home first-aid kit, the first-aid kit in your car, in your suitcase and in other areas where emergencies are likely to occur. The American Academy of Pediatrics (AAP) offers a CPR and first-aid chart. You can order a copy by sending a check for $2.95 to the AAP, Attention: Publications, P.O. Box 747, Elk Grove Village, Illinois, 60009-0747.

A list of emergency numbers should be available beside every phone in the house. Children should be taught to dial 911 in an emergency.

When calling 911, speak slowly and clearly and provide the following information:
- Your first and last name and phone number
- Full address including identifying landmarks
- What happened
- What is being done
- How the child is now
- Ask for emergency instructions.
- Stay on the line until the 911 dispatcher tells you to hang up.

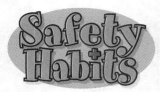

# Choking Alert

*Enroll anyone who cares for your child (including babysitters and grandparents) in a CPR course – training must include CPR for infants.*

Prevent choking by doing the following:

- Do not allow children younger than 5 to have foods listed in the Choking Hazards Health Alert in the *Nutrition* section. Nuts should not be given to children until age 7.

- Keep toys with small parts and small household items out of reach of infants and young children. Pay attention to choking hazard warnings on toy packaging.

  Dangerous household items:

  - Latex balloons
  - Coins
  - Marbles
  - Small toy parts
  - Pen or marker caps
  - Button-type batteries
  - Toys that could be squeezed into a child's mouth

- Cut food for infants and young children and encourage them to chew well.

- Insist that children eat at the table or sitting down. Do not allow children to walk, run, or play with food in their mouths.

- Supervise mealtime for infants and young children.

- Do not allow children to drink from styrofoam cups.

- Use only one-piece pacifiers.

- Keep purses and jewelry boxes out of reach.

Source: American Academy of Pediatrics

# Falls

Falls are the leading cause of injury in children. Babies fall from changing tables. Toddlers fall out of high chairs. Preschoolers fall out of bed. School-age kids fall on the playground. Teenagers fall during athletic activities. Your job as a parent is to protect your child. You won't be able to protect your child from all falls, but you must do everything possible to protect your child from serious falls. Check every area every time for hazards. Don't fall down on your job of preventing falls. No exceptions! No excuses! No regrets!

## The Size of the Problem Nationwide

- Each year, more than 2.5 million children are injured in falls. Children ages 4 and under account for more than half of these injuries.

- Among children ages 4 and under, more than 80 percent of the falls occur at home.

- In 1998, almost 13,000 infants (between 5 months and 15 months) were injured in baby walker-related falls. In 76 percent of baby walker injuries, babies fell down stairs.

- Each year, about 5,000 children (mostly toddlers) are injured by falling from windows. The majority of these falls result in head injuries.

- Each year, more than 230,000 children ages 14 and under are injured in playground-related falls. School-age children, ages 5-14, account for 70 percent of these injuries.

- In 1998, more than 12,000 children were injured in falls from bleachers.

Source: National SAFE KIDS Campaign

# Protective Surfaces

Every 2-1/2 minutes, a child is injured on a playground. Most of these injuries occur when children fall off swings, monkey bars, climbers, or slides. Falls account for 90 percent of the most severe injuries on playgrounds.

The surface under and around the playground equipment makes a big difference in the severity of the injury from a fall. Safer surfaces include: sand (10 inches deep), wood chips (12 inches deep), rubber outdoor mat (follow manufacturer's instructions). Sand and wood chips should be raked weekly to prevent them from packing. The playground surfacing should cover the area surrounding the equipment as follows:

*Swings:* 6 feet on each side of the swing set and two times the height of the swing set in front and back.

*Monkey bars and climbers:* a minimum of 6 feet in every direction.

*Slides under 4 feet high:* a minimum of 6 feet from end of slide.

*Slides more than 4 feet high:* the height of the slide plus 4 feet from the end of slide.

Sources: American Academy of Pediatrics and Kids Health by the Nemours Foundation

# Falls

## Protect Your Child from Falls

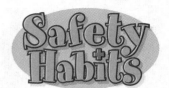

*Prevent falls from furniture/child care products:*

- Don't leave babies alone on beds, changing tables and sofas.
- Always strap your child into the high chair or stroller.
- When your child can sit alone, place crib mattress in a lower position. Move mattress to lowest position when child can get to standing position.
- Never use baby walkers on wheels.
- Pad sharp edges of furniture, especially coffee tables.

*Prevent falls from high places:*

- Never leave a child alone on a balcony, fire escape, or high porch.

*Prevent falls from windows:*

- Move beds, chairs and other furniture away from windows.
- Do not rely on screens to protect a child.
- Do not allow children to play around windows or patio doors.
- Install window guards or keep windows closed to protect children.

*Prevent falls on stairs:*

- Place safety gates at the top and bottom of stairs to protect children under 2.
- Keep stairs clear of clothes, toys, etc.
- Keep doors leading to basement or attic locked.
- Make sure handrails are sturdy and secure. Check regularly for loose posts.

## Prevent falls on the playground:

- Supervise young children on swing sets, slides, and other playground equipment.
- Avoid playgrounds with asphalt, concrete, grass and soil surfaces.

## Prevent falls on slippery surfaces:

- Beware: the bathroom and kitchen are the most common rooms for falls.
- Immediately mop up any water on the floor.
- Use a rubber mat in the bathtub.
- Use throw rugs with nonskid backings.
- Consider installing nonskid stair runners.

## Prevent falls from shopping carts:

- Always strap your child into the seat. Do not use a cart without a safety strap.
- Do not allow your child to ride in the part of the cart where the groceries are placed.
- Do not allow your child to stand in the cart.
- Do not leave your child alone or move more than an arm's length from the cart.

## Prevent falls on escalators:

- Make sure your child always holds onto handrails.
- Do not allow your child to lean against the side panels or sit on the escalator steps.
- Keep your child's hands, feet and clothing away from moving parts and side panels.
- Do not allow your child to run or play on escalator.
- Do not allow your child to walk down the "up" escalator or up the "down" escalator.
- Use an elevator, not an escalator, for a child in a stroller.

# Firearm Safety

Gun safety is for everyone. Many parents delay talking to children about unpleasant subjects like "good touch/bad touch" and gun safety until the child is "old enough." But old enough may not be soon enough. A preschooler is old enough to learn the rules.

Firearm ownership is a fact of life in about half of the homes in the United States. Even if you don't own a gun, your child will be in homes where guns are kept. All children must know what to do if they find a gun – just like they know what to do if they find matches or a lighter.

The rules are simple. Never touch or play with a gun. Leave the room. Tell an adult. Teach preschoolers safety rules by using "what-if" games. Repeat the safety rule several times, and then ask your child a "what-if" question. A gun safety "what-if" might be: "What if you found a gun on the table at Tommy's house? What would you do?" The child uses the rule to answer the question.

Preschoolers like "what-if" games. They like to get the answer right, and they like to hear you praise them for their right answers. "What-if" games allow your child to stay safe from danger in an imaginary world so he or she knows how to stay safe from danger in the real world. Children who learn safety rules early have all the advantages. Safety rules become safety habits. These safety habits prepare children for the years ahead when they must take personal responsibility for their own safety.

# The Size of the Problem Nationwide

- Each year, about 1,500 children ages 14 and under suffer unintentional firearm-related injuries.

- In 1997, almost 150 children ages 14 and under died from unintentional firearm-related injuries. Children ages 10 to 14 accounted for 85 percent of the deaths.

- About 3.3 million children live in homes with firearms that are always or sometimes kept loaded and unlocked.

- Gun locks and load indicators could prevent more than 30 percent of all unintentional firearm deaths.

Source: National SAFE KIDS Campaign

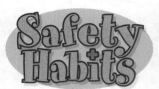

# Protect Your Child from Firearm Injuries

A home where a gun is kept is a dangerous place for children. If you have a gun in your home, it is your responsibility to reduce the risk of firearm injury to children by keeping it unloaded and locking it up. Bullets should be locked up and stored separately from the gun. Make sure children can't get to the keys. Buy and use trigger locks.

Even if you don't keep a gun in your home, your child should know what to do if he or she finds a gun. Teach your child never to touch or play with a gun, to leave the room immediately and to tell an adult.

Be sure your child knows the difference between TV violence and real world violence. Teach your child nonviolent ways to deal with anger and conflict.

# Fire Safety

Fire safety habits go with you everywhere. At home you would never leave matches or a lighter within the reach of children, but that's just where they may be at the home of a smoker or in a motel room. Look for and remove fire hazards when you enter a room. You can do grandparents a favor when you visit by making sure their smoke detectors are in working order. If your family is spending the night away from home, keep children under 5 near you so that in case of a fire, you can take them to safety. With older children, go over fire escape plans from sleeping rooms and agree on a place outside to meet. Never allow your child to sleep in a room without two exits. Never get too busy visiting with friends or relatives to check on children at least once every 30 minutes. Fire safety habits go with you everywhere. No exceptions! No excuses! No regrets!

## Useful Info

## Fire Safety and Your Child with Special Needs

If you have a child with special needs, talk to your doctor, therapist and/or local fire department about your home fire escape plan and how to get your child to safety quickly. To learn about products that can assist you in fire safety planning for your child with special needs, contact Riley Hospital's Community Education Department at 317-274-2964.

# The Size of the Problem Nationwide

- U.S. fire departments respond to one home fire every 70 seconds.

- Each year, almost 50,000 children ages 14 and younger are injured in home fires. More than half of these children are 4 years or younger.

- Home fires caused by children are the leading cause of fire-related death and injury among children ages 9 and under.

- Home fires started by children are most likely to start in the bedroom or living room and areas where children are left alone to play.

- Nearly 80 percent of the home fires started by children are caused by children using matches or lighters to "play with fire."

- A working smoke alarm doubles the chance of surviving a fire.

- Fire-related deaths are three times more likely from smoke inhalation or toxic gases than from heat injury.

- In a typical home fire, you have only two minutes to escape from the house. The need for speed makes an escape plan necessary.

Source: National SAFE KIDS Campaign

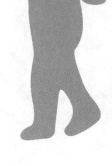

# Fire Safety

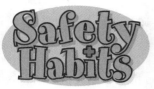

## Protect Your Child from Home Fires

*Install smoke alarms outside all sleeping areas and on all levels of your home.*

## Prevent home fires caused by children by removing fire hazards and setting house rules for fire safety.

**Younger children:**

- Remove hazards: Store matches, lighters and flammable liquids out of reach, preferably in a locked area.

- Fire safety rule: If you find a lighter or match, do not touch. Tell an adult immediately.

- Fire safety rule: Never play with fire.

**Older children:**

- Fire safety rule: No smoking. No incense burning or lighted candles allowed in the bedroom or in any room unless an adult is present.

## Make and practice a home fire escape plan.

- When the alarm sounds, family members should leave home immediately.

- Identify and practice two escape paths from each room. Stress the need for speed in leaving and never returning to a burning building.

- Agree on a spot outside where the family will meet.

- Practice the escape plan at least twice a year. It is wise to have one nighttime practice drill since nighttime fires are common.

## Younger children:

- Practice a fire escape plan using your smoke alarm to signal the drill. In addition, discuss common fears.

- Make sure young children understand not to be afraid of or to hide from the firefighter. Show them pictures of firefighters dressed in firefighting gear or take them on a tour of your local fire station. Teach young children not to hide in closets or under beds.

## Older children:

- Practice a fire escape plan using your smoke alarm to signal the drill. In addition, review the following potential problems:

  - If clothing catches on fire, do not run. Stop, drop and roll.

  - If smoke alarm sounds, leave the house immediately. Test doors before opening them by kneeling at the door, reaching up as high as possible and touching the door, the knob and the space between the door and the frame with the back of your hand. If the door is warm, use another escape route. If the door is cool, open it slowly. Be prepared to slam the door shut if smoke or heat rushes in.

  - If you must escape through smoke, crawl on your hands and knees to the exit. Keep your head low to the floor.

  - If you cannot escape safely, stuff the crack under the door with clothes or a towel to keep smoke out. Go to the window to call for help.

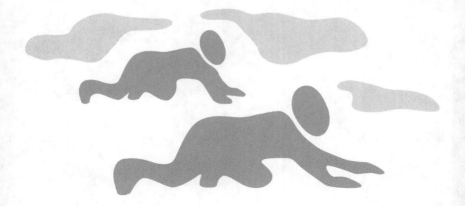

*Attention all parents: The majority of all injuries and deaths from injury in children ages 14 and under occurs in or around the home.*

# The Size of the Problem Nationwide

- In 1998, almost 2,000 children ages 14 and under died from home-related unintentional injuries.

- Each year, almost 4.5 million children ages 14 and under are treated for home-related unintentional injuries.

- Children ages 4 and under suffer the majority of all fatal and nonfatal injuries in the home.

- Every week, one infant or toddler dies by drowning in a bucket.

- Children ages 5 to 14 account for 75 percent of the deaths from firearm injuries.

Source: American Academy of Pediatrics

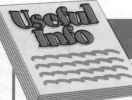

# Who's at Risk?

## Death

| | Cause | Age (Years) |
|---|---|---|
| #1 | Fires and burns | 4 and under |
| #2 | Drowning | 4 and under |
| #3 | Suffocation | 4 and under |
| #4 | Choking | 4 and under |
| #5 | Firearms | 5-14 |
| #6 | Poisoning* | 4 and under |
| #7 | Falls | 4 and under |

*Carbon monoxide is the cause of almost half of all the deaths from poisoning.

## Injuries

| | Cause | Age (Years) |
|---|---|---|
| #1 | Falls | 4 and under |
| | – Stairs | 4 and under |
| | – Furniture | 4 and under |
| | – Windows | 4 and under |
| #2 | Poisoning | 6 and under |
| | – Kitchen • cleaning products | 6 and under |
| | – Bathroom • medications | 6 and under |
| #3 | Burns | 4 and under |
| | – Kitchen • scald (cooking pan) | 4 and under |
| | – Bathroom • scald (bathtub) | 4 and under |

Source: American Academy of Pediatrics

# Home Safety

## Home Safety Checklist

*In our home, every adult and mature child knows:*

- CPR, including infant CPR (see "Be Ready to Rescue" on Choking pages of *Child Safety*).
- First aid (see "Be Ready to Rescue" on Choking pages of *Child Safety*).

*In our home, every adult and mature child knows how to get out. Seconds count!*

- Know and practice home fire escape plan (see "Safety Habits" on Fire Safety pages of *Child Safety*).
- Post fire escape plan by every phone (see "Safety Habits" on Fire Safety pages of *Child Safety*).

*In our home, every adult and mature child knows how to get help:*

- Emergency numbers are posted by every phone (see "Be Ready to Rescue" on Choking pages of *Child Safety*).
- Children practice emergency phone call.

*In our home, every adult and mature child knows where to find:*

- First-aid kit locked or in locked cabinet (see "Be Ready to Rescue" on Choking pages of *Child Safety*).
- First-aid chart posted at phones and in dangerous areas (see "Be Ready to Rescue" on Choking pages of *Child Safety*).

*In our home, I prevent home hazards by:*

- Setting water heater at 120° F (see "Room-by-Room Checklist" on Home Safety pages of *Child Safety*).
- Having chimney cleaned each fall or spring.
- Having fireplace, furnace, wood-burning stove, and gas appliances vented properly and inspected each spring or fall.

- Checking and throwing out medicines that are outdated.
- Marking glass doors with decals.
- Not leaving light sockets empty in lamps or other fixtures.
- Testing for lead paint if home was built before 1978 (see "Safety Habits" on Poisoning Safety pages of *Child Safety*). Call 1-888-532-3547 for certified inspectors.

*In our home, every adult and mature child uses appropriate safety aids and keeps them in place. I regularly check the batteries and working order of the following items:*

- Smoke detectors (see "Safety Habits" on Fire Safety pages of *Child Safety*).
- Carbon monoxide detectors (see "Safety Habits" on Poison Safety pages of *Child Safety*).
- Electrical outlet covers or plugs (see "Top 12 Safety Aids" of *Child Safety*).
- Safety gates (see "Safety Habits" on Falls pages of *Child Safety*).
- Safety latches (see "Top 12 Safety Aids" of *Child Safety*).
- Corner or edge bumpers (see "Top 12 Safety Aids" of *Child Safety*).

*In our home, every adult and mature child knows to keep home hazards out of sight and out of reach:*

- Guns (see "Safety Habits" on Firearm Safety pages of *Child Safety*).
- Medications (see "Safety Habits" on Poison Safety pages of *Child* Safety).
- Dangerous household products (see "Room-by-Room Checklist: Kitchen and Laundry Room" on Home Safety pages of *Child Safety*).
- Fire hazards (see "Safety Habits" on Fire Safety pages of *Child Safety*).
- Knives (see "Room-by-Room Checklist: Kitchen" on Home Safety pages of *Child Safety*).

*In our home, my child is safe because I purchase safe child furniture:*

- High chair (see "Safety Habits" on Falls pages of *Child Safety*).
- Crib (see "Room-by-Room Checklist: Bedroom" on Home Safety pages of *Child Safety*).
- Playpen (see "Room-by-Room Checklist: Living Room and Family Room" on Home Safety pages of *Child Safety*).
- Walker without wheels (see "Safety Habits" on Falls pages of *Child Safety*).
- Bunk beds (see "Room-by-Room Checklist: Bedroom" on Home Safety pages of *Child Safety*).

# Home Safety

*In our home, my child is safe because I check each room for safety hazards. When my child and I are away from home, I do a room-by-room safety check:*

- Kitchen (see "Room-by-Room Checklist: Kitchen" on Home Safety pages of *Child Safety*).
- Bathroom (see "Room-by-Room Checklist: Bathroom" on Home Safety pages of *Child Safety*).
- Family room (see "Room-by-Room Checklist: Family Room and Living Room" on Home Safety pages of *Child Safety*).
- Bedroom (see "Room-by-Room Checklist: Bedroom" on Home Safety pages of *Child Safety*).
- Stairs (see "Room-by-Room Checklist: Stairs and Hallway" on Home Safety pages of *Child Safety*).
- Garage (see "Room-by-Room Checklist: Garage" on Home Safety pages of *Child Safety*).

*In our home, every adult and mature child practices safety habits:*

- Bike (see "Safety Habits" on Bike Safety pages of *Child Safety*).
- Choking (see "Safety Habits" on Choking pages of *Child Safety*).
- Falls (see "Safety Habits" on Falls pages of *Child Safety*).
- Fire (see "Safety Habits" on Fire Safety pages of *Child Safety*).
- Firearm (see "Safety Habits" on Firearm Safety pages of *Child Safety*).
- Pedestrian (see "Safety Habits" on Pedestrian Safety pages of *Child Safety*).
- Poisoning (see "Safety Habits" on Poisoning Safety pages of *Child Safety*).
- Toys (see "Safety Habits" on Toy Safety pages of *Child Safety*).
- Water (see "Safety Habits" on Water Safety pages of *Child Safety*).

*In our home, every adult and mature child makes no exceptions, no excuses, and has no regrets.*

# Kitchen
## General

- Wipe up food or liquids that might cause falls.
- Store dangerous items, such as plastic bags and cleaning products, in out-of-reach cabinets. Store safe items in lower cabinets or drawers.
- Store garbage in a latched cabinet.
- Do not use refrigerator magnets that are small enough to be choking hazards.
- Do not place infants on kitchen counters.
- Use an appliance latch on the refrigerator door.
- Store safe items for your child's play, such as pots and pans and wooden spoons, in one cabinet.
- Children under 4 should not be in the kitchen when meals are being prepared unless one person is available to watch the child.
- Use a playpen as a safe zone for a young child if the child must be in the kitchen with you.
- Make sure your child's high chair has a wide base to prevent tip overs.
- Always use the safety strap when your child is in the high chair.
- Never leave a child alone while in a high chair.

## Scalds and Burns

- Do not hold a child while you are carrying hot liquids.
- Keep playpens away from the stove.
- Use back burners of the stove first and front burners last.
- Keep hot items away from the edge of the counter or table.
- Turn pot handles inward on the stove.
- Protect burner control knobs with knob covers.
- Keep children away from the oven and hot appliances.
- Keep electrical appliances and electrical cords well away from the edge of the counter.

## Kitchen (continued)

- Never leave a detachable appliance cord plugged into the outlet when it has been disconnected from the appliance.
- Use low microwave settings and mix all food thoroughly after heating. Be sure to test food temperature before feeding.
- Never warm your baby's bottle in the microwave.
- Avoid scald burns by keeping children away from the hot water tap on a drinking water dispenser.

Source: American Academy of Pediatrics. *Injury Prevention and Control for Children and Youth* (1997).

# Bathroom
## General

- Bathroom door should be kept closed when the bathroom is not in use. To prevent a child from entering, use a door knob cover or hook-and-eye latch.
- Be sure your locked bathroom door can be unlocked from the outside.
- Use nonskid bath rugs.
- Use a safety latch on the toilet lid.
- Cover the wastebasket.
- Keep cleaning products and harmful items out of sight and out of reach.
- Keep medications in a locked cabinet or box.

# Electrical Hazards

- Unplug electrical appliances when not in use.
- Keep hair dryers, razors, and electrical curlers unplugged and out of reach of children.
- Do not use electrical appliances around water.
- Install ground fault circuit interrupters.

# Bathtub

- Lower the household water heater thermostat to 120° F. If necessary, install an anti-scald device to keep the water temperature less than 120° F.
- Cold water should be turned on first and turned off last. Separate hot and cold water faucets can be hazardous. It is best to have a single faucet.
- Before placing a child in the tub, test the water temperature.
- Do not leave soap bars or shampoo containers on the side of the tub.
- Tub should be empty of water when not in use.
- For younger infants, use an infant tub.
- Do not leave child under the age of 5 – or older if child has increased risk – alone in the tub or shower.
- Stay with the child during bathing. No interruptions. Ignore the phone.
- Purchase a nonskid bath mat or nonskid decals to prevent a slippery tub.
- Use a protective cover over the tub spout to prevent bumps and burns.

Source: American Academy of Pediatrics. *Injury Prevention and Control for Children and Youth* (1997).

## Living Room and Family Room
### General

- Do not use glass-topped tables.
- Do not place heavy objects within a child's reach.
- Make sure TV, VCR, stereo, and other electronic equipment are out of reach of young children.
- Use a VCR guard on the cassette loader.
- To prevent falls from windows, install window guards or screens or a device that prevents windows from opening more than 4 inches. Do not use on windows that are emergency exits.
- Do not allow children to climb on furniture or play near windows.

### Playpens

- Designate a safe area, such as a playpen, for a young child.
- Be sure playpens have fine mesh sides with openings smaller than 1/4 inch or vertical slats less than 2-3/8 inches apart.
- To prevent playpen sides from collapsing, make sure the playpen is always fully opened and in a locked position.
- To prevent a child from climbing out, never place large toys in the playpen.

### Burns and Electrical Hazards

- Hot light bulbs should be out of reach from young children.
- Make sure fireplaces, radiators, and heaters have protective barriers.
- Do not use space heaters.
- If a space heater must be used, make sure it is not within a child's reach. Turn it off when you are asleep or out of the room. Also, check to be sure it automatically turns off if it is knocked over.

## Infant Walkers

- Do not use an infant walker. A "walker" without wheels can be used as an activity center.

- If you have an infant walker, make sure all stairways are blocked and items are out of reach of small hands. Never leave a walker near a stove, space heater or fireplace. Children in walkers should never be near hot liquids.

- An adult should always be present when a child is in a walker.

- To prevent falls, walkers should be kept away from stairs at all times.

Source: American Academy of Pediatrics. *Injury Prevention and Control for Children and Youth* (1997).

# Bedroom
## General

- Never use infant bean bag cushions.
- Never place infants on an adult bed to sleep.
- Never place an infant on a waterbed.
- Never leave an infant alone on a changing table.
- Always cover the wastebasket in the bedroom. Never place dangerous materials such as latex balloons, small or sharp items or rubber bands in the wastebasket.
- The best toy chest is a basket without a lid. If your toy chest has a lid, check to make sure it has hinges that lock and keep the lid open at any angle. All toy chests with lids should have air holes.

## Toddler Bed

- Place guardrails on toddlers' beds.
- Make sure the bed is a minimum of 2 feet from windows, heating vents, radiators, wall lamps, and drapery or window-blind cords.
- Never use an electric blanket.

## Bedroom (continued)
### Bunk Beds

- Never allow children younger than 6 to sleep in the top bunk.
- To prevent entrapment of the child's head, legs, or arms, add additional boards to the bed frame to close off any space more than 3-1/2 inches between the lower edge of the guardrails and the upper edge of the bed frame.
- Make sure the top and bottom bunk have a guardrail next to the wall and at both ends of the bed. The top bunk should also have a guardrail on the outer side.
- Check to make sure guardrails extend 5 inches above the mattress.
- Make sure the mattress is well secured with cross supports made of wood slats, metal straps or sturdy wires.
- Do not allow children to play on bunk beds.
- Never use an electric blanket.

### Cribs

- Make sure cribs do not have slats that are more than 2-3/8 inches apart.
- Check to make sure the crib does not have splinters or cracks and that lead-free paint was used.
- Never use cribs with corner posts.
- To prevent entrapment of the child's head, legs or arms, never use cribs with decorative cutouts in the headboard.
- Check to make sure there are not crossbars on the sides of the crib.
- When the sides of the crib have been lowered, they should be a minimum of 9 inches above the mattress.
- When the baby is in the crib, always keep the sides up.
- The sides should be operated with a locking, hand-operated latch that is secure from accidental release.

- To prevent entrapment, make sure the mattress is the same size as the crib and that there are no gaps.

- The minimum rail height should be 26 inches from the top of the railing to the mattress when set at the lowest level.

- No pillows, quilts, stuffed animals, sheepskin, or other soft items should be in an infant's bed.

- Make sure your child's crib meets current federal and voluntary industry standards. Do not use older cribs. Use safety tassels for miniblinds. Remove strings from toys and pacifiers.

- Use bumper pads in the crib until your child can stand. Bumper pads can then be removed.

- Lower the crib mattress when the infant is able to sit alone. When the infant can stand, lower the mattress to its lowest position.

- Crib toys should not be strung across the crib. Remove crib toys when the infant begins to push up on hands and knees or when he or she is 5 months old.

- To help prevent a child from climbing out of the crib, never place large toys in the crib.

- Make sure hanging crib toys are not within the child's reach.

- Place a carpet or rug underneath the crib.

- To prevent a child from climbing out of the crib, never place large toys in the crib.

- Never use an electric blanket.

Source: American Academy of Pediatrics. *Injury Prevention and Control for Children and Youth* (1997).

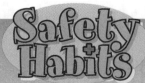

## Checking Out Used Furniture

If you purchase used baby furniture such as a crib or used equipment such as a car seat, check for recall information by checking the Consumer Product Safety Commission Web site at *www.cpsc.gov* or by calling 1-800-638-2772.

Source: American Academy of Pediatrics. *Injury Prevention and Control for Children and Youth* (1997).

# Room-by-Room Checklist

## Halls and Stairways
### General

- Keep stairs clear of toys, clothes, and other objects.
- Make sure banisters are secure. There should be no more than 4 inches between the upright posts.
- Make sure plants are out of reach.
- Use nonskid backing for carpet on the stairs, at the bottom of the stairs and in the hallway.
- Keep toys and other clutter out of the hallway.
- Be careful not to overwax floors.
- Clean up spills immediately.
- Be sure hallways and stairways are well lit.

Source: American Academy of Pediatrics. *Injury Prevention and Control for Children and Youth* (1997).

## Laundry Room
### General

- Do not allow young children in the laundry room.
- Make sure the dryer and washer doors are always closed.
- Make sure dangerous items, such as bleach, detergent and other items, are out of sight and out of reach of children.
- Do not leave water standing in buckets, diaper pails, or other containers.

Source: American Academy of Pediatrics. *Injury Prevention and Control for Children and Youth* (1997).

# Garage
## General

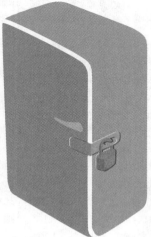

- Make sure tools, chemicals, and equipment are locked away from children. Store chemicals in their original containers.

- Always keep garage door locked. Do not allow children in the garage alone.

- Before driving into or out of the garage, make sure you know where your child is.

- Keep garage freezers locked at all times.

- If you have an automatic garage door opener, make sure it has an auto-reverse feature. Never let children race to beat the door when it is closing.

## Car

- Never leave a young child alone in the car.

- Never let your child play with the car windows (electric or automatic).

- Do not keep cigarette lighters in the car.

- Make sure rear-door child locks are working until the child is at least 6 years old.

- Teach your child to get out of the car on the curb side.

- Make sure the keys are not in the ignition when you are washing or working on the car.

- Never leave a car running in an unventilated area, especially if the garage is attached to the house.

Source: Johns Hopkins Children's Center. *First Aid for Children Fast* (1994).

# Motor Vehicle Safety

Make every ride a safe ride. Don't let things like being on vacation, being in a hurry, being late, or the length of the ride wear you down. Even when you feel too tired to move, transfer your child's safety seat to the car that your infant will be riding in. And, if your own father tries to talk you out of putting your fussing baby in that "awful car seat way back there with nothing to look at" and if he goes on to tell you about that coast-to-coast car trip where you sat happily on your mother's lap in the front seat for the whole trip, don't give in. You know the right thing to do, so do it. Make every ride a safe ride. No exceptions! No excuses! No regrets!

## The Size of the Problem Nationwide

- Motor vehicle crashes are the leading cause of injury-related death in children ages 1 to 14.

- In 1998, almost 300,000 children were injured while riding in a motor vehicle.

- The risk of death and injury in a motor vehicle crash is higher for children under age 4 than for other age groups. About 1 in 3 children in this age group rides unrestrained.

- The proper use of properly installed child safety seats could prevent 70 percent of motor vehicle-related deaths for infants younger than 1 year and more than half of the deaths of children ages 1 to 4.

- The majority of motor vehicle crashes occur within 25 miles of home and on roads with posted speed limits of 40 mph or less.

- Motor vehicle crashes on country roads are more frequent, more severe, and have a higher death rate than crashes on city streets.

Source: National SAFE KIDS Campaign

## Child Safety Seats 101

**Useful Info**

In order to protect young children from injury in a motor vehicle accident, safety features must be designed with the child in mind.

An effective infant restraint system must be able to restrain small and easily broken bones. It must prevent damage to soft and easily injured internal organs. And it must prevent the infant's fairly large and heavy head from rapid movements that strain the neck and spinal cord.

Only by faithfully following the instructions with your child safety seat will your child benefit from the protection the seat was designed to provide.

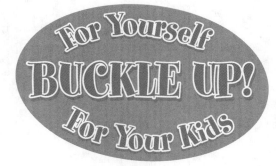

For Yourself BUCKLE UP! For Your Kids

## Motor Vehicle Safety and Your Child with Special Needs

**Health Alert**

If you have a child with special needs or with certain health problems, your child may require special adaptive equipment for safe and comfortable transportation.
There are a number of resources you can use, beginning with the car seat safety program in the hospital where your child was born. You can also call the Automotive Safety for Children Program at Riley Hospital at 1-800-KID-N-CAR.

# Motor Vehicle Safety

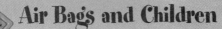

Child Safety

## Air Bags and Children

**Health Alert**

Air bags are dangerous for children younger than age 12. Passenger air bags have caused the death of more than 100 children. Almost all of these children were improperly restrained or unrestrained at the time of the crash.

Air bags only inflate in head-on crashes. They inflate at tremendous speeds of up to 200 mph. The air bag loses air immediately after it inflates.

The likely cause of death with air bag injuries is a head or neck injury caused by a blow to the head from the inflating air bag. The injury to infants in rear-facing safety seats is caused by the inflating bag hitting the back of the infant's seat behind the infant's head.

Source: American Academy of Pediatrics

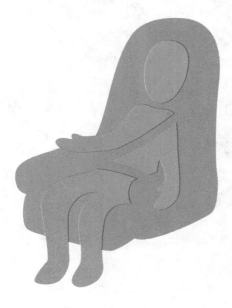

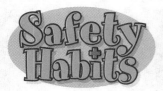

# Protect Your Child from Motor Vehicle Injury

*Infants* should ride in the back seat in rear-facing car seats until they weigh at least 20 pounds and are 1 year old. Infants should never be placed in the front seat with an air bag on the passenger side.

*Children older than 1 year* who weigh between 20 and 40 pounds should ride in the back seat in forward-facing car seats. Children fit in the car seat properly if their ears are below the top of the back of the car seat and their shoulders are below the seat strap slots.

*Children who weigh more than 40 pounds* and are more than 3 feet 4 inches tall (usually under 10 years old) should sit in booster seats. The booster seat is used to make the lap and shoulder belt fit properly. The booster seat must be secured with both the lap and shoulder belt.

*Children who weigh more than 80 pounds* and are more than 4 feet 10 inches tall (usually 10 years or older) are big enough to have the lap and shoulder belts fit correctly. The shoulder belt should never be under the child's arms or behind the child's back. If a child must slouch to sit comfortably with knees bent at the edge of the seat, then the child is not tall enough for the lap and shoulder belt to fit properly.

*All children under 13 years old* should sit in the back seat of the car using the proper restraint system. The back seat is safer than the front seat even if there is no air bag on the passenger side.

Source: American Academy of Pediatrics

# Pedestrian Safety

No exceptions! No excuses! No regrets! Be a good pedestrian safety role model. Most parents are faithful in teaching their children about pedestrian safety. Children are taught to cross at a crosswalk or corner and to obey traffic signals. Children hear what their parents say, but children also see what their parents do. Many parents have a different set of rules for themselves. Parents jaywalk, and parents frequently cross a street with the "Don't Walk" sign blinking. When children hear one thing and see another, safety rules seem more like safety "suggestions." If you want your child to believe that rules are rules and you want your child to follow those rules, then you need to follow the rules. Be a good role model. No exceptions! No excuses! No regrets!

## The Size of the Problem Nationwide

- In 1998, 20,000 children ages 14 and younger were injured when struck by a motor vehicle.

- Almost 1,000 children ages 14 and younger die as a result of being hit by a motor vehicle. About half of all child pedestrian deaths occur between 4 and 8 p.m.

- Pedestrian injury is the second leading cause of injury-related deaths in children ages 5 to 9.

- More than 500 toddlers ages 1 and 2 are killed in pedestrian accidents each year. The majority of these deaths occur when a toddler is struck by a car backing down a driveway.

Source: National SAFE KIDS Campaign

# Pedestrian Safety and the Child with Special Needs

If your child uses a wheelchair on sidewalks or streets, make certain the wheelchair is properly marked with reflective tape or lights. Adding a bike flag to the wheelchair makes it more visible in crowded areas.

# Protect Your Child from Pedestrian Injuries

**Safety Habits**

*Supervise young children.* Do not allow young children to play unsupervised near a street or driveway.

*Do not allow children to play in the street.* Playing in the street, even a neighborhood street that is not busy, is not safe. Do not allow children on wheels – skateboards, scooters, roller blades, bicycles, wheelchairs – to enter a street from a driveway, especially a sloping driveway. This rule applies to children on sleds or snowboards. Teach children never to dart out into the street after a ball or a pet.

*Teach children safety rules for walking.* Cross streets in a straight line at the corner or in crosswalks. Never enter the street between parked cars. Obey traffic signals. Look left-right-left before crossing the street and continue checking as you cross. Walk on sidewalks where possible. On a road with no sidewalk, walk facing oncoming traffic. Wear light-colored clothing or reflective clothing on dark days or at nighttime.

# Poison Safety

Keep poisons out of sight. Keep children in sight. As soon as toddlers learn to walk, curiosity sets their bodies in motion – almost constant motion. Without a microscope or a laboratory, these junior scientists rely on a five-step discovery process. Step 1: See it. Step 2: Get to it. Step 3: Pick it up. Step 4: Shake it, rattle it, and if possible, open it. Step 5: Taste it. Pet food, a candy wrapper, a cigarette butt – if it is within reach, it is fair game. The kitchen, the bathroom, the garage – since the toddler has no sense of safe or unsafe, each room offers endless possibilities. Dishwasher detergent, grandma's heart medicine, turpentine – even if it smells bad or tastes yucky, the toddler puts it through the five-step discovery process. So much to see. So much to taste. Ask any emergency room doctor or the poison control center for other examples that will break your heart. Keep poisons out of sight. Keep children in sight. No exceptions! No excuses! No regrets!

## The Size of the Problem Nationwide

- Every 30 seconds, a childhood poisoning occurs in the United States. In 1998, more than 1.1 million unintentional poisonings among children ages 1 to 5 were reported.

- About 90 percent of poisonings occur in the home. The majority of childhood poisonings occur in children younger than 5.

- Among children 5 and under, 60 percent of poisonings are by household products such as cosmetics, cleaning substances, plants, toys, pesticides, art supplies, and alcohol.

- Among children 4 and younger, about one-third of poisonings by prescription medication involve the grandparent's or great-grandparent's medication.

- Iron or multi-vitamins with iron are responsible for 30 percent of child deaths due to medication poisoning.

Source: National SAFE KIDS Campaign

# Poison Preparedness

Keep the Universal Poison Center number (1-800-222-1222) by every phone in your home. This number will automatically connect you to your local poison center. If you suspect poisoning, call immediately.

Poison control centers manage millions of poisonings a year. Their telephone instructions make it possible for 3 out of every 4 childhood poisonings to be managed at home. These centers prevent about 50,000 hospitalizations and 400,000 trips to doctors' offices each year.

**Keep a bottle of syrup of ipecac on hand for each child in your family. Store syrup of ipecac with your other medicines in a locked closet or cabinet. Do not give syrup of ipecac unless instructed by the poison control center or your doctor.**

Syrup of ipecac is a medication that causes vomiting by irritating the stomach. It is available without a prescription at most pharmacies.

## Useful Info

# Poison Safety and the Child with Special Needs

Some children with special needs continue the toddler's habit of exploring objects by mouthing them. Children who continue to mouth objects are frequently unaware that they are in danger of choking or poisoning.

Every place that your child receives care should be regularly checked for objects that are dangerous. Every person who cares for your child should be aware of the need for increased caution and the importance of keeping items out of reach.

# Poison Safety

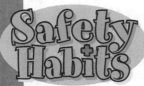

## Protect Your Child from Household Poisons

Store all medications, including vitamins and nonprescription drugs, in a locked closet or cabinet. Return medication to storage immediately after use. Purchase medications with child-resistant safety caps.

Never call medicine "candy." Don't take medication in front of children. Ask all guests to keep their medications out of sight and out of reach of children.

Do not store medications and household products with food.

Store alcoholic beverages and the following household products out of reach, preferably under lock: cleaning fluids, detergents, bleaches, insect spray, weed killer, fertilizer, gasoline, car wax, and turpentine. Store all products in their original containers.

# Lead Poisoning

- About 900,000 children ages 1 to 5 have blood lead levels high enough to cause problems with growth, development and intelligence.

- The most common cause of lead poisoning among children is dust from lead-based paint.

Source: National SAFE KIDS Campaign

# Protect Your Child from Lead Poisoning

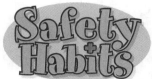

Ask your doctor about blood lead screening if your child lives in or regularly visits a house or child care facility built before 1950 or a home built before 1978 that is being remodeled or has been remodeled in the last 6 months.

Also check with your doctor if your child has a sibling or playmate who has or had a high blood lead level.

Source: American Academy of Pediatrics

# Carbon Monoxide Poisoning

- In 1998, more than 2,000 children ages 5 and younger were treated for carbon monoxide poisoning.

- Each year, nearly 30 children ages 14 and younger die from carbon monoxide poisoning.

Source: National SAFE KIDS Campaign

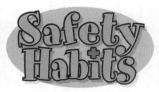

# Protect Your Child from Carbon Monoxide Poisoning

Install carbon monoxide alarms near bedrooms and on each floor of your home. Make sure that space heaters, furnaces, fireplaces, and wood-burning stoves are properly vented and inspected each year.

# Toy Safety

Take safety warning signs on toy packaging very seriously. When you read "not recommended for children under 3" on a toy package, the Consumer Product Safety Commission (CPSC) wants you to know that the toy is not considered safe for a normally developing child under 3. The problem may be that the toy is not safe for a child under 3 because of its small size or loose parts. Or the problem may be that a child under 3 doesn't have the coordination to play with the toy safely, doesn't understand the risks of unsafe play, or doesn't have the self-control to follow the rules for safe play. The safety warning covers a lot of territory. Think carefully before you ignore it.

## The Size of the Problem Nationwide

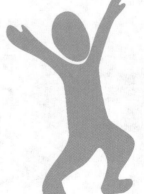

- In 1998, more than 120,000 children ages 14 and younger were treated for toy-related injuries. Sixty percent of these injuries occurred in children 4 and younger.

- Sixty percent of toy-related deaths are caused by choking. Latex balloons account for half of these deaths.

- The majority of toy-related injuries are caused by riding toys (primarily wagons and tricycles).

- In 1998, almost 11,000 children ages 14 and younger were injured with BB guns and pellet guns.

Source: National SAFE KIDS Campaign

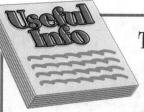

# The Toy Safety Story

The safety of more than 3 billion toys sold each year should be of concern to parents. However, it's doubtful that most parents pause very long to think about the potential hazards of the toy at the top of the "most wanted" list. Fortunately, there are several groups that are concerned with toy safety.

The U.S. Consumer Product Safety Commission (CPSC), created by Congress in 1972, is a regulatory agency that monitors toy-related injuries, sets safety standards, issues product recalls and provides public education. The CPSC has authority over 15,000 consumer products, for example, toys, bicycles, cribs, etc. *To report a toy-related injury or toy hazard, call the toll-free hotline at 800-638-2772.*

The American Society for Testing and Materials (ASTM), established in 1986, is a nonprofit organization that sets standards for safety, establishes guidelines for safety testing, and sets design guidelines for toy manufacturers.

# Protect Your Child from BB Gun and Pellet Gun Injury

BB guns and pellet guns are not toys. BB guns, pellet guns and air rifles are also called nonpowder firearms. Consumer Product Safety Commission (CPSC) warning labels say, "Not a toy." "Adult supervision required." CPSC warns against children under 16 years of age using these guns.

Toy guns that shoot small objects into the air are also dangerous.

Caution! Toy guns can be mistaken for real guns in dim light.

# Toy Safety

## Protect Your Child from Toy-Related Injuries

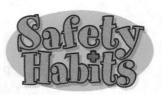

Choose your child's toys carefully (see "Tips for Buying Safe Toys").

Supervise your child's play. Do not allow your child to play close to dangerous areas, such as swimming pools, stairways, and busy streets. Never allow a child of any age to play with uninflated or broken balloons. Stop reckless, rough, or dangerous play immediately. Do not allow your child to play with a toy intended for an older child. Keep all toys with small parts away from children under 5.

Store toys properly. Store toys on the shelf or in a toy chest. Older children's toys should be kept separate from the toys of younger children. Never store a toy in its original packing. Teach your child to pick up and put toys away.

Keep toys in good condition. Make it a habit to look for damaged or broken parts that may present a hazard. Never leave metal toys outside overnight. If you are concerned about a toy's safety, use this rule: "If in doubt, throw it out."

Source: American Academy of Pediatrics

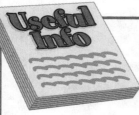

# Tips for Buying Safe Toys

*Look for a toy that matches the interest, developmental age, and the skills of the child. When purchasing a toy, be sure:* the toy is constructed with safety in mind, the intended owner will use the toy safely, and the toy is not a safety hazard for younger siblings in the family. Refer to these safety tips before you buy.

- Pay attention to the safety warning on the toy package.

- Include essential safety gear as part of a gift, for example, bike and helmet.

- Think large. Avoid toys small enough to put into a child's mouth. Make sure there are no removable parts.

- Avoid toys that shoot small objects.

- Avoid toys that make loud or shrill noises. Sounds may be too loud for your child's sensitive hearing.

- Look for sturdy toy construction.

- Watch out for sharp points or edges and toys made from thin plastic.

- Avoid toys that could cause poisoning such as paint sets and crayons (unless labeled as nontoxic) and small batteries.

- Do not buy hobby kits or chemistry sets for a child under 12 years.

- Buy only "UL*approved" electric toys.

- Choose a toy chest carefully. The best toy chest is a box or basket without a lid. If the chest has a hinged lid, make sure it has a lid support that will hold the lid open in any position. The chest should have ventilation holes. The edges should be smooth. The finish should be nontoxic.

*UL (Underwriters Laboratories Inc.)
Source: American Academy of Pediatrics

# Water Safety

Watch out for kids around water. Whether the water is in a puddle, a bucket, a bathtub, a wading pool, your neighbor's pool or the ocean, watch out for kids around water. Water is a "kid magnet." It attracts and entertains. But watch out for kids around water. Water is the second leading cause of injury-related deaths in children 14 and younger. Drowning is quick and quiet. Swimmers and nonswimmers drown, babies and teenagers drown. Watch out for kids around water. No exceptions! No excuses! No regrets!

## The Size of the Problem Nationwide

- Drowning is the leading cause of injury-related death among children ages 1 to 4 and the second leading cause of death for children 14 and younger.

- For children under age 1, more than half of the drownings occur in the bathtub. Children this age also drown in toilets and buckets.

- For children ages 1 to 4, swimming pools account for 9 out of 10 drownings.

- For children ages 5 to 14, swimming pools and open water, such as lakes and rivers, account for most drownings.

- Among adolescent boys, alcohol is the major contributing factor in half of the drownings.

- When drownings and near-drownings in the United States are averaged over an entire year, 40 children die each week, 115 are hospitalized, and 12 suffer severe brain damage. The cost of care for a near-drowning victim with brain damage can be more than $4.5 million.

Source: National SAFE KIDS Campaign

# Facts about Drowning

Drownings and near-drownings typically occur when a child is left unsupervised for a brief period of time. Most children who drown in home swimming pools were inside the house when last seen by the parents and had been out of the parents' sight for less than five minutes.

Most people are unaware that children may not make noise or splash frantically when they get into trouble in the water. Drowning frequently happens quickly and silently. Two minutes after a child goes under water, the child becomes unconscious. After four to six minutes, brain damage is likely.

Children who are discovered within the first several minutes have the highest rate of survival. Most children found after 10 minutes and who require CPR for longer than 25 minutes do not survive.

Source: National SAFE KIDS Campaign

# Be Ready to Rescue!

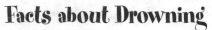

If you own a pool, live near a pond, lake or river, or love water sports, you should know CPR (cardiopulmonary resuscitation).

Your training should include rescue techniques for both adults and children. Courses are available through the American Red Cross, the American Heart Association, your local hospital and the fire department.

In case of an emergency, you should also have written CPR instructions and rescue equipment, such as a shepherd's hook, safety ring and rope, nearby. A telephone to call for help should also be available.

# Water Safety

## Swimming Lessons

Formal swimming lessons are not recommended for children until after their 4th birthday. Swimming requires developmental abilities that children under 4 do not yet have. The American Academy of Pediatrics also warns parents that children younger than 4 are at risk of swallowing too much water or picking up infection from dirty water.

Even after swimming lessons, parents should never assume a child is safe in water. A child who accidentally swims into deep water may get confused, then panic and drown. Children need to be watched at all times in the water. Children should never swim alone.

# Protect Your Child from Drowning

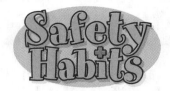

*Water safety tips for children under 1:*

- Empty all buckets and any other large containers after use.

- Keep the bathroom door closed at all times.

- Never leave a child alone in the bathroom.

- Keep toilets closed or use toilet latches.

- Use a rigid, lockable cover on a hot tub, spa, or whirlpool.

- In addition, follow the safety tips listed below.

*Water safety tips for all children:*

- Children in the water should be supervised at all times.

- Empty wading pools after each use.

- Inflatable pool toys should never be used to keep a child afloat.

- Never allow running or pushing in pool areas.

- Children should never swim alone.

- Do not allow children to chew gum or eat while swimming, diving, or playing in the water.

- Do not allow diving if there is more than one person on the board.

- Never dive into an above-ground pool.

- Never swim during thunder or lightning.

- Young children should always wear a life jacket while in a boat or playing around water.

- Children 4 and older should be enrolled in swimming classes taught by an accredited instructor.

- Teach teenagers about the dangers of drinking alcohol and swimming, boating, or water skiing.

Source: National SAFE KIDS Campaign

# Resources

## Organizations
### General Safety

*The American Academy of Pediatrics*
141 Northwest Point Boulevard
P.O. Box 747
Elk Grove Village, Illinois 60009-0747
800-433-9016 (phone)
847-434-8000 (fax)
www.arp.org

*American Red Cross (ARC) National Headquarters*
430 17th Street NW
Washington, D.C. 20006
202-639-3685 (or call the local chapter)
www.redcross.org
Provides information on a wide variety of safety instruction
materials and cardiopulmonary resuscitation (CPR) classes.

*Consumer Product Safety Commission*
4330 East-West Highway
Bethesda, Maryland 20814-4408
800-638-2772
www.cpsc.gov

*Indiana SAFE KIDS Coalition*
575 West Drive, Room 004
Indianapolis, Indiana 46202
317-278-3218
888-832-3219

*National Center for Injury Prevention and Control*
Mailstop K65
4770 Buford Highway N.E.
Atlanta, Georgia 30341-3724
770-488-1506 (phone)
770-488-1667 (fax)
www.cdc.gov/ncipc/cmprfact.htm

*National SAFE KIDS Campaign*
1301 Pennsylvania Avenue
Suite 1000
Washington, D.C. 20004
202-662-0600
www.safekids.org

*Riley Hospital Community Education Department*
Riley Hospital for Children
575 West Drive, Room 008
Indianapolis, Indiana 46202-5272
317-274-2964
www.rileyforkids.org
Provides information and educational resources on child health, safety and advocacy.

*SAFE USA*
P.O. Box 8189
Silver Springs, Maryland 20907-8189
888-252-7751
www.cdc.gov/safeusa

## Automotive Safety

*Automotive Safety for Children Program*
Riley Hospital for Children
575 West Drive, Room 004
Indianapolis, Indiana 46202
317-274-2977
Provides material and reference information on the transportation and occupant protection of children, including children with special needs.

## Bicycle Safety

*Consumer Product Safety Commission*
4330 East-West Highway
Bethesda, Maryland 20814-4408
800-638-2772
www.cpsc.gov
www.bikehelmet.org
Provides bike helmet information for parents and activities for kids.

# Resources

## Child Abuse

*Childhelp USA*
*National Child Abuse Hotline*
15757 North 78th Street
Scottsdale, Arizona 85260
800-422-4453
Provides comprehensive crisis counseling by mental health professionals for adult and child victims of child abuse and neglect, offenders and parents who are fearful that they will abuse, and parents who want information on how to be effective parents.

## Child Care

*Safe Sitter, Inc.*
5670 Caito Drive #172
Indianapolis, Indiana 46226
317-543-3840
800-255-4089
317-545-SAFE (7233) (fax)
www.safesitter.org
Provides referral to Safe Sitter teaching sites and safety education for babysitters and parents.

## Drug and Alcohol Safety

*National Clearinghouse for Alcohol and Drug Information (NCADI)*
P.O. Box 2345
Rockville, Maryland 20847-2345
800-729-6686
www.health.org
Provides a variety of government publications about the prevention of drug use by children.

## PRIDE Youth Programs
4684 S. Evergreen
Newaygo, MI 49337
800-668-9277 (phone)
231-652-4400 (fax)
www.prideyouthprograms.org
A national resource center that can provide prevention services in the area of alcohol and other drugs.

## Partnership for a Drug-Free America
405 Lexington Avenue
Suite 1601
New York, New York 10174
212-922-1560
www.drugfreeamerica.org
Provides free information about various drugs and tips to help your kids stay away from them.

## Fire Safety

### National Fire Protection Association
617-984-7826
www.nfpa.org
www.sparky.org
Provides free packet on fire safety and additional fire safety tips.

## Food Safety

### United States Department of Agriculture
### U.S. Agriculture Department Meat and Poultry Hotline
800-535-4555
www.USDA.gov
Home economists, registered dietitians and food technologists answer questions about food safety weekdays from 10 a.m. to 4 p.m. (EST). Recorded information is available 24 hours.

# Resources

## Missing Children

*National Center for Missing and Exploited Children (NCMEC)*
699 Prince Street
Arlington, Virginia 22314
703-235-3900
800-843-5678 (hotline)
www.ncmec.org
To report a suspicion of child abuse or the sighting of a missing child or to report a child who is missing.

## Playground Safety

*Consumer Product Safety Commission*
4330 East-West Highway
Bethesda, Maryland 20814-4408
800-638-2772
www.cpsc.gov
Provides *Handbook for Public Playground Safety* as well as other safety tips.

*The National Program for Playground Safety*
800-554-PLAY (800-554-7529)
www.uni.edu/playground

## Poison Safety

*Universal Poison Center Number*
800-222-1222
This number will automatically connect you to your local poison center.

## Recalled Products

*Consumer Product Safety Commission*
4330 East-West Highway
Bethesda, Maryland 20814-4408
800-638-2772
www.cpsc.gov

*Kids in Danger*
www.kidsindanger.org
Provides information and educates parents about product recalls.

# Recommended Books

*Child Safe: A Practical Guide to Preventing Childhood Injuries*
By Mark A Brandenburg, M.D. (2000). Three Rivers Press.

*The Complete Idiot's Guide to Child Safety*
By Miriam Bachar Settle, Ph.D., and Susan Crites Price. (2000).
Alpha Books.

# Web Sites for Parents and Kids

*Consumer Product Safety Commission*
www.cpsc.gov/kids/bb.html

*Kids Health for Parents*
www.kidshealth.org

*National Fire Protection Association*
www.nfpa.org
www.sparky.org (family Web site)

*Riley Hospital Community Education Department*
www.rileyforkids.org

*Safe Sitter*
www.safesitter.org

# Resources

## Online Child Safety Stores
## (Contact These Companies for Free Catalogs)

*Baby Guard*
703-821-1231
www.babyguard.com

*Baby Protectors*
800-859-0657
www.babypro.com

*Safe Beginnings*
800-598-8911
www.safebeginnings.com

*The Child Safety Company*
800-708-1648
www.childsafety.com

# Index

# Emergency Information

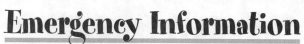

Our Home Address

_____

Our Phone Number

_____

## EMERGENCY SERVICES

EMS

_____

Police

_____

Fire

_____

Poison Center

**1-800-222-1222**

## HEALTH SERVICES

Child's Doctor

_____

Pharmacy

_____

24-Hour Pharmacy

_____

Child's Dentist

_____

## IF PARENT CANNOT BE REACHED IN AN EMERGENCY, CALL

Family Member

_____

Neighbor

_____

Locked first-aid kit is located

_____

Key is located

_____